English for Nursing, Academic Skills

Susan Dandridge Bosher

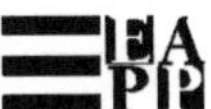

MICHIGAN SERIES IN ENGLISH FOR
ACADEMIC & PROFESSIONAL PURPOSES
Series Editors: John M. Swales & Christine B. Feak

Ann Arbor
The University of Michigan Press

Published in the United States of America
The University of Michigan Press
Manufactured in the United States of America

Printed on acid-free paper

ISBN-13: 978-0-472-03227-3

2011 2010 2009 2008 4 3 2 1

Dedication

To Habib, Reshad, Lyla, and Ariana
Without your love and support,
this project would never have been completed.

Contents

Acknowledgments

I am grateful to the many nursing colleagues who have given so generously of their time and expertise over the years to educate me about the profession of nursing and who have contributed in so many ways to the development of the English for Cross-Cultural Nursing course that I have taught at the College of St. Catherine since 2000. Many of the materials developed for that course have been revised and included in this textbook on academic skills and in the textbook to follow on clinical skills.

A special thanks to Alice Swan, Suellen Campbell, and Pamela Hamre for their unwavering support to leveling the playing field in nursing education for students of diverse cultural and linguistic backgrounds; to the many nursing faculty who welcomed me into their lectures, labs, and clinicals; to Deborah Anderson for her lecture and lecture outline on mental health and illness; to many other nursing faculty for their feedback and insights about the many ways in which nurses and nursing students use language and cultural knowledge in their work; to the many immigrant and international nursing students for their feedback and insights about language and culture-related skills and tasks in nursing that are the most challenging for them; to the many pre-nursing ESL students for their feedback and critique of materials and activities developed; and to Beth Koenig for her enthusiastic support and helpful suggestions along the way.

Many thanks also to the U.S. Department of Health and Human Services Multicultural Nursing Education Opportunities Grant for funding to conduct the initial needs analysis of ESL nursing students in the baccalaureate degree program (Bosher, 2001a, 2001b, 2006); to the College of St. Catherine for their support of a year-long sabbatical to write; and to the Archibald Bush Foundation Diversity and Democracy Grant for funding to complete the project. Thanks, too, to Christine Diaz for her skillful transcription of the lecture and to Kirsten Walters for her careful attention to the details of grant funding.

Grateful acknowledgment is given to the following authors, publishers, and individuals for permission to reprint previously published materials:

BMJ Publishing Group for "Mental Health and Vietnamese Refugees" from the *Western Journal of Medicine*, © 1992. Reprinted with permission of BMJ Publishing, Inc.

Suzanne Gordon for "Nurse, Interrupted," *The American Prospect*, Volume 11, Number 7: February 14, 2000. The American Prospect, 2000 L Street NW, Suite 717, Washington, DC 20036. Reprinted with permission. All rights reserved.

Kozier, Barbara J.; Erb, Glenora; Berman, Audrey J; Snyder, Shirlee, FUNDAMENTALS OF NURSING: CONCEPTS, PROCEDURES, & PRACTICES, and FUNDAMENTALS CARD PKG., 7th Edition, © 2004. Reprinted with permission of Pearson Education.

Massachusetts Medical Society for "Nursing in the Crossfire" from *The New England Journal of Medicine.* Copyright 2002 Massachusetts Medical Society. All rights reserved.

Mother Jones for "Caring Means Curing" © 1992. Reprinted with permission.

SAGE Publications for excerpt and relevant references from "The Evolution of a Crisis" by Bobbi Kimball and Edward O'Neil in *Policy, Politics & Nursing Practice.* © 2001. Reprinted with permission of SAGE Publications, Inc., and "Review of Literature on Culture and Pain of Adults with Focus on Mexican-Americans" in *Journal of Transnational Nursing* © 1991. Reprinted with permission of SAGE Publications, Inc.

Wiley-Blackwell Publishing Ltd. for "Nurses' perceptions of sexuality relating to patient care" by Caitrian Guthrie in the *Journal of Clinical Nursing.* © 1999*;* and "West African beliefs about mental illness" by Ann Hales in *Perspectives in Psychiatric Care.* © 1996. Reprinted with permission.

Wiley for "Current Nursing Practice Related to Sexuality" © 1993. Reprinted with permission.

For voice talent, Pat Grimes.

Every effort has been made to contact the copyright holders for permission to reprint borrowed material. We regret any oversight that may have occurred and will rectify them in future printings of the book.

Introduction

This textbook is one of two *English for Nursing* textbooks designed to prepare non-native speakers of English for the language-related skills and tasks and cultural content necessary for success in associate- and baccalaureate-degree nursing programs in the United States. The textbook could also be used in re-entry programs in nursing for internationally educated nurses who need to familiarize themselves with nursing in the United States. This book focuses on **academic** strategies and skills for nursing, including reading and vocabulary, research and writing, and listening and note-taking.

Essential to students' success in nursing courses are the ability to: read and understand nursing textbooks and articles from nursing journals; listen carefully to lectures and take accurate notes; participate in class and group discussions; think critically; and do well on multiple-choice tests. Students must also be able to write coherent, well-organized papers; to analyze, synthesize, and integrate information from a variety of outside sources; and follow academic conventions of paraphrasing, summarizing, quoting, and documenting.

Students must also be aware of and develop strategies for handling issues in nursing that, from a cultural perspective, they may not be comfortable with because nursing in the United States is based on certain cultural values, beliefs, and practices that may or may not be consistent with students' own values, beliefs, and practices. Working through such issues as mental health and illness, and sexuality in nursing, before students enter nursing programs will not only increase students' degree of comfort and confidence in addressing these issues in their courses, but also their ability to handle these issues in practice.

To address these many objectives, this book is divided into six units, each of which focuses on a different academic skill taught through nursing content. The nursing content focuses on nursing as a profession, the nursing shortage, the role of culture in nursing, and culturally sensitive topics in nursing such as mental illness and death and dying. The content is presented in each unit through two readings, either articles from nursing journals or chapters from nursing textbooks. Each unit includes activities based on the academic skills introduced, as well as discussion questions and writing assignments that are more communicative in nature. Available online (*www.press.umich.edu/esl/nursingacad/*) is a lecture on mental health and illness so students can practice the listening and note-taking skills necessary for lecture comprehension. Available for teachers online is the Instructor's Manual, which provides supplementary material and exercises on grammar and vocabulary points, quizzes for some of the units, and a transcript of the lecture. An answer key is also available online for exercises in the textbook.

The audience for this textbook is ESL pre-nursing students, at both the baccalaureate and associate-degree levels and at the intermediate to advanced levels of language proficiency. Students should be working toward admission to an associate- or baccalaureate-degree program in nursing and should have already taken general academic ESL classes.

The textbook is equally appropriate for immigrants (whether recently arrived, long-term residents, or citizens) and international students. It is also appropriate for internationally educated nurses who need to strengthen their language skills and/or familiarize themselves with cultural issues in nursing while preparing to enter the U.S. workforce.

UNIT 1

Reading Skills for Nursing

The **content-based objectives** include learning about

- Nursing as a profession, from both a historical and contemporary perspective
- Essential characteristics of nursing, in particular the role of caring and the importance of trust
- Responsibilities of a nurse
- The role of nursing in innovative practices in health care

The **skill-based objectives** include

- Pre-reading strategies
  - activating prior knowledge about a topic
  - previewing a reading for organizational features
- Basic reading skills
  - skimming for an overview of a reading
  - scanning for specific information
- Reading strategies
  - making predictions about content
  - underlining main points
  - writing marginal notes
  - predicting test questions
- Vocabulary strategy
  - using contextual clues

At the end of the unit, you will reflect on your definition and understanding of nursing in the United States.

Pre-Reading Strategies

To help you get the most out of the reading you will do as a nursing student, try one of these two pre-reading activities or strategies:

- **Activate prior knowledge** about the topic.
- **Preview the reading** for organizational features.

Activating Prior Knowledge about a Topic

When you encounter new information, it is helpful to first consider what you already know about the topic. It is also helpful to explore any thoughts and feelings you might have about it. The topic of this unit is What Is Nursing? To activate prior knowledge on this topic, think about and answer these questions.

1. What is nursing?
2. What types of qualifications or skills do you think nurses need? Make a list.
3. What experiences have you had with nurses or nursing in the United States?

Previewing a Reading

It is also often helpful to consider the many organizational features and resources for learning that are often included in a reading, particularly in textbooks. These features can include any combination of the following: title, subtitle, abstract, objectives, vocabulary list, headings and subheadings, excerpts from the text, bulleted items or lists, words in **bold** type, words in *italics,* photographs and other figures, graphs and charts, tables, boxes, research notes, summary, review questions, links to other chapters, links to media resources, suggested readings, Internet resources, and reference list.

Previewing a reading introduces you to everything that has been provided to support your learning or reading. In a textbook the same organizational features are usually provided in every unit, so carefully previewing the first unit will also introduce you to the organizational features of every unit in the textbook.

"Historical and Contemporary Nursing Practice" is the title of the first chapter in a widely used nursing textbook called *Fundamentals of Nursing—Concepts, Process, and Practice* by Kozier, Erb, Berman, and Snyder (2004c). The chapter provides an introduction to the profession of nursing, both from a historical and contemporary perspective. Obtain a copy of this chapter or a similar one from a textbook used in the nursing program at your college or university. Portions of the chapter from Kozier et al. (2004c) are reprinted on pages 6–12, as Reading 1.1.

Preview the chapter, identifying its organizational features and resources, and answer the questions.

1. Check the organizational features that are included in the nursing textbook chapter:

_____ Title

_____ Subtitle

_____ Abstract

_____ Objectives (referred to as: ______________________________)

_____ Vocabulary list (referred to as: __________________________)

_____ Headings and subheadings

_____ Excerpts from the text, highlighted in some way (e.g., in **bold** type)

_____ Bulleted items or lists

_____ Words in **bold** type

_____ Words in *italics*

_____ Photographs

_____ Graphs and charts

_____ Tables

_____ Boxes

_____ Research notes

_____ Summary (referred to as: ______________________________)

_____ Review questions

_____ Links to other chapters

_____ Links to media resources (e.g., CD-ROM or companion website)

_____ Suggested readings

_____ Related research

_____ Internet resources

_____ Reference list

_____ Selected bibliography

_____ Other: ____

Heading and subheadings are used to organize information from general to specific levels. The first heading in a chapter is at the most general level. Subheadings are formatted differently from headings. Find the headings and subheadings in Reading 1.1. Answer the questions.

2. How many levels of headings and subheadings are there? ___________

   What formatting differences do you notice? ____________________

   ____

3. How many headings (not subheadings) are there? ___________
   List them:

   ____

   ____

   ____

   ____

   ____

   ____

   ____

Reading Skills and Strategies

We read in different ways, depending on our purpose. If you want an overview or general information about a reading, you **skim** it. If you want to locate specific information, you **scan** it. If you are reading for a deeper understanding, you might use various strategies that help you identify and learn the main points: **making predictions**, **underlining main points, writing marginal notes,** and **predicting test questions**.

Skimming: Getting an Overview of a Reading

Getting an overview of a reading is like looking at a map of a city you are visiting for the first time, to see where all the important places are located. The most efficient way to get an overview of a reading is by skimming or reading portions of it. If what you are reading has an **abstract,** read that first. An abstract is the paragraph located at the beginning of an article, before the actual article itself, that gives a brief summary of the contents of the article.

To skim, read the introduction section or the first paragraph of the article. Then, read the headings and subheadings. Read the first paragraph after each new heading and the first sentence after each new subheading. Look at any figures and tables, and read the titles. Finally, read the concluding section of the article or the last paragraph.

Preview Reading 1.1. Then read the excerpt of the first chapter of Kozier et al. (2004c) as instructed by your teacher (Reading 1.1). Notice that it consists of the introduction to the chapter, the first paragraph after each new heading, the first sentence after each new subheading, and the concluding section to the chapter/highlights.

Reading 1.1

Historical and Contemporary Nursing Practice*

Barbara Kozier, MN, RN; Glenora Erb, BSN, RN;
Audrey Berman, PhD, RN, AOCN; Shirlee J. Snyder, EdD, RN

Learning Outcomes

After completing this chapter, you will be able to:

- Discuss historical and contemporary factors influencing the development of nursing.
- Identify the essential aspects of nursing.
- Identify four major areas within the scope of nursing practice.
- Identify the purposes of nurse practice acts and standards for nursing practice.
- Describe the roles of nurses.
- Describe the expanded career roles and their functions.
- Discuss the criteria of a profession and the professionalization of nursing.
- Discuss Benner's levels of nursing proficiency.
- Relate essential nursing values to attitudes, personal qualities, and professional behaviors.
- Explain the functions of national and international nurses' associations.

Nursing today is far different from nursing as it was practiced years ago, and it is expected to continue changing during the 21st century. To comprehend present-day nursing and at the same time prepare for the future, one must understand not only past events but also contemporary nursing practice and the sociological and historical factors that affect it.

Historical Perspectives

Nursing has undergone dramatic change in response to societal needs and influences. A look at nursing's beginnings reveals its continuing struggle for autonomy and professionalization. In recent decades, a renewed interest in nursing history has produced a growing amount of related literature. This section highlights selected aspects of events that have influenced nursing practice. Recurring themes of women's roles and status, religious values, war, societal attitudes, and visionary nursing leadership have influenced nursing practice in the past. Many of these factors still exert their influence today.

Women's Roles

Traditional female roles of wife, mother, daughter, and sister have always included the care and nurturing of other family members.

* From Kozier, Barbara; Erb, Glenora; Berman, Audrey J.; Snyder, Shirlee, FUNDAMENTALS OF NURSING: CONCEPTS, PROCEDURES, & PRACTICES, 7th Edition, © 2004. Reprinted by permission of Pearson Education, Inc., Upper Saddle River, NJ.

Religion

Religion has also played a significant role in the development of nursing.

War

Throughout history, wars have accentuated the need for nurses.

Societal Attitudes

Society's attitudes about nurses and nursing have significantly influenced professional nursing.

Nursing Leaders

Florence Nightingale, Clara Barton, Lillian Wald, Lavinia Dock, Margaret Sanger, and Mary Breckinridge are among the leaders who have made notable contributions both to nursing's history and to women's history.

Contemporary Nursing Practice

An understanding of contemporary nursing practice includes a look at definitions of nursing, recipients of nursing, scope of nursing, settings for nursing practice, nurse practice acts, and current standards of clinical nursing practice.

Definitions of Nursing

Florence Nightingale defined nursing over 100 years ago as "the act of utilizing the environment of the patient to assist him in his recovery" (Nightingale, 1860).[1]

Recipients of Nursing

The recipients of nursing are sometimes called consumers, sometimes patients, and sometimes clients.

Scope of Nursing

Nurses provide care for three types of clients: individuals, families, and communities.

Promoting Health and Wellness
Wellness is a state of well-being.

Preventing Illness
The goal of illness prevention programs is to maintain optimal health by preventing disease.

Restoring Health
Restoring health focuses on the ill client and it extends from early detection of disease through helping the client during the recovery period.

Care of the Dying
This area of nursing practice involves comforting and caring for people of all ages who are dying.

[1]Nightingale, F. (1969). *Notes on nursing: What it is, and what it is not.* New York: Dover (original work published 1860).

Settings for Nursing

In the past, the acute care hospital was the main practice setting open to most nurses.

Nurse Practice Acts

Nurse practice acts, or legal acts for professional nursing practice, regulate the practice of nursing in the United States and Canada.

Standards of Clinical Nursing Practice

Establishing and implementing standards of practice are major functions of a professional organization.

Roles and Functions of the Nurse

Nurses assume a number of roles when they provide care to clients. Nurses often carry out these roles concurrently, not exclusively of one another. For example, the nurse may act as a counselor while providing physical care and teaching aspects of that care. The roles required at a specific time depend on the needs of the client and aspects of the particular environment.

Caregiver

The caregiver role has traditionally included those activities that assist the client physically and psychologically while preserving the client's dignity.

Communicator

Communication is integral to all nursing roles.

Teacher

As a teacher, the nurse helps clients learn about their health and the health care procedures they need to perform to restore or maintain their health.

Client Advocate

A client advocate acts to protect the client.

Counselor

Counseling is the process of helping a client to recognize and cope with stressful psychological or social problems, to develop improved interpersonal relationships, and to promote personal growth.

Change Agent

The nurse acts as a change agent when assisting others, that is, clients, to make modifications in their own behavior.

Leader

A leader influences others to work together to accomplish a specific goal.

Manager

The nurse manages the nursing care of individuals, families, and communities.

Case Manager

Nurse case managers work with the multidisciplinary health care team to measure the effectiveness of the case management plan and to monitor outcomes.

Research Consumer

Nurses often use research to improve client care.

Expanded Career Roles

Nurses are fulfilling expanded career roles, such as those of nurse practitioner, clinical nurse specialist, nurse midwife, nurse educator, nurse researcher, and nurse anesthetist, all of which allow greater independence and autonomy.

Criteria of a Profession

Nursing is gaining recognition as a profession. Profession has been defined as an occupation that requires extensive education or a calling that requires special knowledge, skill, and preparation. A profession is generally distinguished from other kinds of occupations by (a) its requirement of prolonged, specialized training to acquire a body of knowledge pertinent to the role to be performed; (b) an orientation of the individual toward service, either to a community or to an organization; (c) ongoing research; (d) code of ethics; (e) autonomy; and (f) professional organization.

Specialized Education

Specialized education is an important aspect of professional status.

Body of Knowledge

As a profession, nursing is establishing a well-defined body of knowledge and expertise.

Service Orientation

A service orientation differentiates nursing from an occupation pursued primarily for profit.

Ongoing Research

Increasing research in nursing is contributing to nursing practice.

Code of Ethics

Nurses have traditionally placed a high value on the worth and dignity of others.

Autonomy

A profession is autonomous if it regulates itself and sets standards for its members.

Professional Organization

Operation under the umbrella of a professional organization differentiates a profession from an occupation.

Socialization to Nursing

The standards of education and practice for the profession are determined by the members of the profession, rather than by outsiders. The education of the professional involves a complete socialization process, more far reaching in its social and attitudinal aspects and its technical features than is usually required in other kinds of occupations.

Critical Values of Nursing

It is within the nursing educational program that the nurse develops, clarifies, and internalizes professional values.

Factors Influencing Contemporary Nursing Practice

To understand nursing as it is practiced today and as it will be practiced tomorrow requires an understanding of some of the social forces currently influencing this profession. These forces usually affect the entire health care system, and nursing, as a major component of that system, cannot avoid the effects.

Economics

Greater financial support provided through public and private health insurance programs has increased the demand for nursing care.

Consumer Demands

Consumers of nursing services (the public) have become an increasingly effective force in changing nursing practice.

Family Structure

New family structures are influencing the need for and provision of nursing services.

Science and Technology

Advances in science and technology affect nursing practice.

Information and Telecommunications

The Information Superhighway or Internet has already impacted health care, with more and more clients becoming well informed about their health concerns.

Legislation

Legislation about nursing practice and health matters affects both the public and nursing. Changes in legislation relating to health also affect nursing.

Demography

Demography is the study of population, including statistics about distribution by age and place of residence, mortality (death), and morbidity (incidence of disease).

The New Nursing Shortage

Multiple factors influence the new nursing shortage and these factors contribute to the current nursing shortage being different from previous shortages.

Collective Bargaining

More nurses are using collective bargaining to deal with their concerns.

Nursing Associations

Professional nursing associations have provided leadership that affects many areas of nursing.

Nursing Organizations

As nursing has developed, an increasing number of nursing organizations have formed. These organizations are at the local, state, national, and international levels. The organizations that involve most North American nurses are the American Nurses Association, the Canadian Nurses Association, the National League for Nursing, the International Council of Nurses, and the National Student Nurses' Association. The number of nursing specialty organizations is also increasing, for example, the Academy of Medical Surgical Nursing, the American Association of Nurse Anesthetists, and the National Black Nurses Association. Participation in the activities of nursing associations enhances the growth of involved individuals and helps nurses collectively influence policies affecting nursing practice.

Chapter Highlights

- Historical perspectives of nursing practice reveal recurring themes or influencing factors. For example, women have traditionally cared for others, but often in subservient roles. Religious orders left an imprint on nursing by instilling such values as compassion, devotion to duty, and hard work. Wars created an increased need for nurses and medical specialties. Societal attitudes have influenced nursing's image. Visionary leaders have made notable contributions to improve the status of nursing.
- The scope of nursing practice includes promoting wellness, preventing illness, restoring health, and care of the dying.
- Although traditionally the majority of nurses were employed in hospital settings, today the numbers of nurses working in home health care, ambulatory care, and community health settings are increasing.
- Nurse practice acts vary among states and nurses are responsible for knowing the act that governs their practice.
- Standards of clinical nursing practice provide criteria against which the effectiveness of nursing care and professional performance behaviors can be evaluated.
- Every nurse may function in a variety of roles that are not exclusive of one another; in reality, they often occur together and serve to clarify the nurse's activities. These roles include caregiver, communicator, teacher, client advocate, counselor, change agent, leader, manager, case manager, and research consumer.
- With advanced education and experience, nurses can fulfill advanced practice roles such as clinical nurse specialist, nurse practitioner, nurse midwife, nurse anesthetist, educator, administrator, and researcher.
- A desired goal of nursing is professionalism, which necessitates specialized education; a unique body of knowledge, including specific skills and abilities; ongoing research; a code of ethics; autonomy; a service orientation; and a professional organization.
- Socialization is a lifelong process by which people become functioning participants of a society or a group. It is a reciprocal learning process that is brought about by interaction with other people and established boundaries of behavior. Socialization to professional nursing practice is the process whereby the values and norms of the nursing profession are internalized into the nurse's own behavior and self-concept. The nurse acquires the knowledge, skill, and attitudes characteristic of the profession.
- Although several models of the socialization process have been developed, Benner's five stages of novice, advanced beginner, competent, proficient, and expert may serve as guidelines to establish the phase and extent of an individual's socialization.
- Contemporary nursing practice is influenced by economics, changing demands for nurses, consumer demand, family structure, science and technology, information and telecommunications, legislation, demographic and social changes, the new nursing shortage, collective bargaining, and the work of nursing associations.
- Participation in the activities of nursing associations enhances the growth of involved individuals and helps nurses collectively influence policies that affect nursing practice.

Predicting Content

When you skim a reading to get an overview, you are, in part, predicting content. When you get an overview of a reading, you get an idea of what you will learn and what to look for when you read. It helps you evaluate information, make inferences, and make connections; in short, it helps you to become engaged in the reading.

Now that you have read Reading 1.1, write ten questions about nursing that you think will be answered or ten topics that you think will be discussed in the reading.

Scanning: Looking for Specific Information

Scanning also involves looking at the reading but this time for specific information. The information could be located anywhere in the text—in the abstract or in the title of a figure or table. To scan, create an image in your mind of the word, phrase, concept, or piece of information you are looking for, and move your eyes quickly over the reading until you locate the same image in the reading.

Underlining

One strategy to help reading new material is to underline or use a highlighter to identify the main points. Underlining can help you identify what is most important in an article and should be reviewed for a test at a later time.

In textbooks, main points are often provided for the reader in objectives or learning outcomes at the beginning of a chapter and/or in a summary or highlights provided at the end. In addition, important points in textbooks are often found in the **topic** (or first) **sentences** of paragraphs. Determining the main points is more complicated in readings that do not provide the organizational features that are included in nursing textbooks or that do not follow a linear organization from the introduction, to the body, to the conclusion. In these articles, you can identify the main points by looking for general statements that are presented as statements of truth, analysis, or evaluation. Main points are supported by other, more specific points, details, and/or examples.

For example, in Reading 1.2, "Caring Means Curing" on pages 18–22, the first main point of the article does not appear until Paragraph 6 in the sentence: "Janet Craig . . . embodies the relationship between caring and curing that is at the heart of nursing" (page 18). The first five paragraphs describe an "hour of intense activity" for Janet Craig, an intensive care nurse. According to the author, the heart of nursing is the relationship between caring and curing. This is a main point. It is a general statement, supported by the preceding five-paragraph description of how Janet Craig attends not just to the complex physical needs of her patients, but to their emotional needs, as well.

Writing Marginal Notes

Writing while you read can help you learn the material. Making notes in the margins of a reading is one way of writing while you read; taking notes on a separate sheet of paper is another. There are different types of marginal notes. Some notes turn a main point into a phrase. (See Figure 1.) These notes are guides to a reading. Later, when you review for a test, these notes can help you locate the main points. You don't have to re-read the entire chapter or article; you can review your marginal notes and then select specific sections that you need to re-read. Obviously, if the book is not yours, you should not write in it.

Another type of marginal note is a question. These can be questions about main points, or they can be questions about points you don't understand or that you don't agree with. Ask your teacher for help on the questions later. By turning main points into questions, you are already preparing for the next test. You are anticipating questions that will be on the test.

Read the entire chapter "Historical and Contemporary Nursing Practice," paying particular attention to sections that correspond to or give you information about one of the learning outcomes listed on page 6. Underline or highlight main points, and write notes in the margins to identify or ask questions about the main points.

Predicting Test Questions

You are preparing for a test by predicting test questions. With nursing textbooks, use the objectives listed at the beginning of a chapter and turn each one into a test question. When you later answer these questions, you are reviewing the corresponding points in the chapter.

Write questions based on the Learning Outcomes for Reading 1.1 on page 6. First, familiarize yourself with the Learning Outcomes and the Chapter Highlights. Re-write each learning outcome as a test question.

1. Number the Learning Outcomes at the beginning of the chapter. Then, turn to the Chapter Highlights at the end. For each chapter highlight, write the number of the corresponding learning outcome.

   ### Example
   Learning Outcome 1 (Discuss historical . . . factors influencing the development of nursing) corresponds with Chapter Highlight 1 (Historical perspectives of nursing practice reveal recurring themes or influencing factors. . .). Write 1 next to the first chapter highlight.
   Note: There may not be a chapter highlight for every learning outcome, or vice versa.

Figure 1 Reading Strategies: Underlining and Writing Marginal Notes

8 UNIT 1/The Nature of Nursing

themes common to defs. of nursing

- Nursing is a science.
- Nursing is client centered.
- Nursing is holistic.
- Nursing is adaptive.
- Nursing is concerned with health promotion, health maintenance, and health restoration.
- Nursing is a helping profession.

ANA def. of nrsng / *chngs to def.* / *Obj. #2*

Professional nursing associations have also examined nursing and developed their definitions of it. In 1973, the American Nurses Association (ANA) described nursing practice as "direct, goal oriented, and adaptable to the needs of the individual, the family, and community during health and illness" (ANA, 1973, p. 2). In 1980, the ANA changed this definition of nursing to this: "Nursing is the diagnosis and treatment of human responses of actual or potential health problems" (ANA 1980, p. 9). In 1995, the ANA recognized the influence and contribution of the science of caring to nursing philosophy and practice. Their most recent definition of nursing acknowledges four essential features of contemporary nursing practice:

4 essen. aspects of nrsng

- Attention to the full range of human experiences and responses to health and illness without restriction to a problem-focused orientation
- Integration of objective data with knowledge gained from an understanding of the client or group's subjective experience
- Application of scientific knowledge to the processes of diagnosis and treatment
- Provision of a caring relationship that facilitates health and healing (ANA, 1995)

imp. of caring

Research to explore the meaning of caring in nursing has been increasing. For example, Sherwood (1997) conducted a meta-synthesis of qualitative studies describing caring from the perspective of clients. Likewise, Beck (2001) analyzed qualitative studies that researched caring within schools of nursing. Details about caring are discussed in Chapter 24.

def. of consumer

Recipients of Nursing

The recipients of nursing are sometimes called consumers, sometimes patients, and sometimes clients. A **consumer** is an individual, a group of people, or a community that uses a service or commodity. People who use health care products or services are consumers of health care.

def. of patient / *prob. with term "patient"*

A patient is a person who is waiting for or undergoing medical treatment and care. The word *patient* comes from a Latin word meaning "to suffer" or "to bear." Traditionally, the person "receiving health care has been called a patient. Usually, people become patients when they seek assistance because of illness or for surgery. Some nurses believe that the word patient implies passive acceptance of the decisions and care of health professionals. Additionally, with the emphasis on health promotion and prevention of illness, many recipients of nursing care are not ill. Moreover, nurses interact with family members and significant others to provide support, information, and comfort in addition to caring for the patient.

client = preferred term / *def. of client* / *resp. for own health*

For these reasons, nurses increasingly refer to recipients of health care as *clients.* A client is a person who engages the advice or services of another who is qualified to provide this service. The term *client* presents the receivers of health care as collaborators in the care, that is, as people who are also responsible for their own health. Thus, the health status of a client is the responsibility of the individual in collaboration with health professionals. In this book, *client* is the preferred term, although *consumer* and *patient* are used in some instances.

3 types of clients

Scope of Nursing

Nurses provide care for three types of clients: individuals, families, and communities. Theoretical frameworks applicable to these client types, as well as assessments of individual, family, and community health are discussed in detail in Chapter 12.

4 areas of nrsng practice / *Obj. #3*

Nursing practice involves four areas: promoting health and wellness, preventing illness, restoring health, and care of the dying.

def. of wellness / *ex.*

① Promoting Health and Wellness

Wellness is a state of well-being. It means engaging in attitudes and behavior that enhance the quality of life and maximize personal potential (Anspaugh, Hamrick, & Rosata, 2001). Nurses promote wellness in clients who are both healthy and ill. This may involve individual and community activities to enhance healthy lifestyles, such as improving nutrition and physical fitness, preventing drug and alcohol misuse, restricting smoking, and preventing accidents and injury in the home and workplace.

goal = maintain optimal health / *exs.*

② Preventing Illness

The goal of illness prevention programs is to maintain optimal health by preventing disease. Nursing activities that prevent illness include immunizations, prenatal and infant care, and prevention of sexually transmitted disease.

focuses on ill client / *nrsng actv. to restore health* / *exs.*

③ Restoring Health

Restoring health focuses on the ill client and it extend from early detection of disease through helping the client during the recovery period. Nursing activities include the following:

- Providing direct care to the ill person, such as administering medications, baths, and specific procedures and treatments
- Performing diagnostic and assessment procedures such as measuring blood pressure and examining feces for occult blood
- Consulting with other health care professionals about client problem
- Teaching clients about recovery activities, such as exercise that will accelerate recovery after a stroke
- Rehabilitating clients to their optimal functional level following physical or mental illness, injury, or chemical addiction

comfort and care for dying / *help support persons cope* / *hospice*

④ Care of the Dying

This area of nursing practice involves comforting and caring for people of all ages who are dying. It includes helping client live as comfortably as possible until death and helping support persons cope with death. Nurses carrying out these activities work in homes, hospitals, and extended care facilities. Some agencies, called *hospices,* are specifically designed for this purpose.

Adapted from Kozier et al., 2004c, p. 8.

2. Write at least one question for each of the ten learning outcomes. The answers to these questions should consist of the information contained in the corresponding chapter highlight(s). The first one has been done for you.

   Example
   Questions for Outcome 1, "Discuss historical and contemporary factors influencing the development of nursing," are:

   1a. Historically, what are some important factors that have influenced the development of nursing?
   1b. What are some important, contemporary factors that influence the profession of nursing today?

   Note that the answers to these two questions give you the information contained in the first chapter highlight and the next-to-last highlight.

3. Locate the answer to each of your ten questions from Kozier et al. (2004c). Write the number of the learning outcome in the margin.

If you have completed all of the activities in this unit, reviewing for a test or quiz should be relatively easy. Answer the questions you have written for the activity on predicting test questions, and look back in the complete chapter in Kozier et al. (2004c) to help you. Write your questions and answers on notecards, with questions on one side and answers on the other. Re-read the sections in the textbook you have underlined, especially those parts that relate to learning objectives, and review your marginal notes. If you have time, skim through the entire chapter again.

Memorizing information for nursing tests is usually not helpful as nursing tests generally ask you to apply information in new ways. (See Unit 2 for discussion of critical reading skills.)

Another Perspective on Nursing

Reading 1.2, "Caring Means Curing," was written by Suzanne Gordon, an author and journalist, who has written many books and articles about nursing for the popular press. This article was first published in a magazine, not a nursing journal. It was written for the average person who does not have specialized knowledge or training in the field of nursing. Through a series of stories, Gordon illustrates the work of nurses and the vital role they play in patient care. She describes a variety of innovative new practices in health care, such as primary nursing and collaborative physician/nurse care of patients, and she advocates for a more visible role and greater responsibilities for nurses in health care.

Skim through Reading 1.2. Read the title and subtitle. Read the first and last paragraphs and the topic sentence of every paragraph in between. Predict what you think the article is about. Write five questions that you think will be answered in the reading.

As you read, underline or highlight the main points. In addition, write notes in the margins to help you identify and learn what is most important in the reading and quickly locate that information at a later time. Words that have been selected for vocabulary work (see page 33) are in bold type.

Reading 1.2

Caring Means Curing

Suzanne Gordon, BA, is an author and journalist in Boston, Massachusetts.

An expanded role for nurses would bring healthy results to our medical system

In the **pediatric intensive care unit** at the University of California San Francisco (UCSF) Medical Center, four nurses are clustered around the bed of an unconscious 7-year-old Cambodian boy who was hit by a truck several days earlier. A plastic **respirator tube** snakes out of his mouth, and other tubes and wires connect him to **intravenous drips, evacuation bags,** and a series of **monitors** that provide second-by-second displays of his heart and **respiratory rhythms.** His right leg, bent at the knee, is held up **in traction.** His face is so swollen that a visitor finds it hard to look too closely. He is **sedated** to shield him from pain and to prevent him from injuring himself.

A small, slight woman in a white uniform stands at the boy's bedside, talking to two of the nurses. Janet Craig, a nurse educator based in the pediatric intensive care unit, is questioning her colleagues about the boy's progress and their efforts to care for him. In addition to purely medical questions, she asks, "Can we get a picture of him before the accident, so we can see what he looks like, and measure his progress?"

She turns to her left, where two small, tense Cambodian women—the patient's mother, who does not speak English, and a relative who can translate for her—keep an anxious **bedside vigil**. Craig wants to find out about the boy's favorite music, pictures, and books. "It would be good if he can hear some music and see some familiar pictures when we wake him up," she tells the women. And then the three discuss how they will keep the normally active boy quiet and entertained during what will be a long hospital stay.

As they talk, a sudden commotion diverts Craig's attention. A nurse approaches and whispers in her ear. Craig rushes toward the room of another patient, hastily explaining that this 17-year-old girl has been a frequent visitor to the intensive care unit. She was born with a **congenital heart defect** that has required a number of surgeries, and recently she may have **suffered** a **heart attack.** Five days earlier, when surgeons opened her up, they found so much damage that they **implanted** a permanent **pacemaker.** They also decided she would need a heart transplant to survive over the long term.

Moments ago, she began having **chest pains,** and the unit immediately went into action. Now the girl, attached to an **EKG** and other **diagnostic** equipment, lies on the bed, clutching a Snoopy doll and looking frightened. While doctors and nurses evaluate and respond to her physical **symptoms,** Janet Craig is working on another diagnosis—a **nursing diagnosis**—of the girl's emotional needs. Craig concentrates on reducing her patient's anxiety about both her condition and the **high-tech treatment** she is receiving. She sees that the girl is becoming very **agitated** and that this might **aggravate** her condition. So she tries to calm and reassure her, explaining what the doctors and nurses are doing and why. She remains with the patient until the **cardiologist** determines that she is not having a heart attack.

In this hour of intense activity, and in the time she spends each day attending to complex cases like these, Janet Craig, an intensive care nurse for 14 years, embodies the relationship between caring and curing that is at the heart of nursing. In hospitals and in the community, nurses are the ones who help treat not only patients' complex physical needs but their interlinked emotional needs as well. While doctors focus on limb, heart, or lung, nurses carry out the medical regimens that physicians prescribe, as well as monitoring intricate human needs.

Attending to the human dimension of disease is far more than a feminine nicety. It is vital to the patient's survival. "Among other things," says Patricia Benner, professor of **physiological nursing** at UCSF and coauthor of *The Primacy of Caring,* "a nurse's job is to make sure hospitals don't scare patients to death."

Health care has always been a collaboration between care and cure, and health-care institutions have always depended on a marriage between medicine, a profession until recently entirely male-dominated, and nursing, still 97 percent female. Like most conjugal relationships in patriarchal societies, this one has silenced the voice and obscured the contributions of the female partner. Throughout this [20th] century, Americans have been taught to equate health care with medical care and to believe that physicians do all of the curing and even a great deal of the caring.

Although most media reports about health rely almost exclusively on physicians or medical researchers for insight, analysis, and information, in contemporary America it is the nurses who do a great deal of the curing and caring. They outnumber doctors by about three to one: around 1.7 million registered nurses to 575,000 physicians. Nurses are the backbone of hospitals, where 70 percent of them work. During an average **hospital stay** of five days, a patient might spend less than an hour with his or her physician.

Nurses take care of patients 24 hours a day, seven days a week. If a patient with a broken leg complains of chest pain, it's the nurse who will contact the physician about a suspected **pulmonary embolism.** If a patient with **metastatic breast cancer** comes in for **chemotherapy** and complains of dizziness, shivering, and simply not feeling like herself, the nurse will alert the **oncologist** to the possibility that the cancer has traveled to the brain.

In addition to following physicians' treatment plans, nurses establish treatment plans of their own. They **assess** patients' basic needs and do for them what they cannot do alone; they help educate people about how to **cope** with a disease or the aftermath of **surgery;** they become deeply involved—as **patient advocates**—in helping patients and families make informed decisions about major surgery and **termination** of **life-support systems.**

All of these responsibilities should make nurses major participants in the evolving debate about national health care. Yet to most of the public and policymakers, they remain virtually invisible.

When 29-year-old Betsy Gemmell, a **primary nurse** at Boston's Beth Israel Hospital, comes to work, she is hardly invisible. She graduated from Simmons College with a combined degree in nursing and women's studies and decided to take a job at Beth Israel because of its nationally recognized commitment to nursing. The hospital's nurse in chief, Joyce Clifford, has long promoted the idea of "primary nursing": Just as a patient has a doctor whose name he or she knows, so, too, should the patient have a primary nurse. This nurse draws up a **nursing plan** for her patients, and other nurses follow that plan when she is off duty. Patients admitted more than once will be admitted, whenever possible, to the floor on which their primary nurse is practicing.

At 7:30 each morning, Gemmell sees her first patient, who today is a 68-year-old woman **propped up** in her bed. She smiles welcomingly when Gemmell comes in. A grandmother now, she developed major **circulatory** problems in her legs when she was having her own children. For decades, she's suffered from **recurring ulcers** on her legs, and she has had several **operations** and long **hospitalizations.**

Gemmell asks how she slept and makes sure the **bedridden** woman has had no trouble with breakfast. Then she checks her **vital signs—temperature, blood pressure, heart** and **respiratory rate**—and examines the area around the **point of entry** of her intravenous tube for any sign of infection.

Later in the day, Gemmell comes in to talk with this patient again and change her **dressing.** The woman's legs are **mottled** and red with a tough, almost leathery shell; they seem like scarred veterans of a prolonged, relentless battle. Under the bandages, a large weeping ulcer needs to be cleaned with **saline solution,** and, while she cleans it, Gemmell judges how well the **tissue** is healing. While she unwraps, dabs gingerly, and rewraps, the woman watches intently, wincing occasionally.

Gemmell explains everything she is doing and discovering. This forthright communication is a result of the relationship she has established with her patient during previous long hospital stays. "Not only have I worked to get to know her, but she has responded to that effort and now knows and trusts me," Gemmell says proudly. Trust, she points out, has been crucial. Before the woman came in for her first hospitalization, Gemmell remembers, she was terrified. She had delayed coming to the doctor because she was afraid of a long stay, and even more afraid that she would lose her leg. This delay, in fact, may have contributed to the long hospitalization that she feared.

"Because we worked so hard with her, she came in sooner during the second **episode,**" reports Gemmell, who notes that this sort of case is typical. "We see a lot of patients for a long time, and this relational work is crucial in getting them to a better state of health. We know that, if we deal with them as people, we're better able to assess their response to an illness and help them either heal or cope."

While many people—including many physicians—ignore the importance of nursing work, nurses are trying to demonstrate that a health-care system that truly encourages physician-nurse collaboration will significantly improve patient care. On Betsy Gemmell's unit at Beth Israel Hospital, Seven North, this kind of teamwork is not only encouraged but also studied.

Seven North's collaborative care unit is largely the creation of Adele Pike, a **clinical nurse specialist** who was convinced that integrating physician and nursing treatment plans and improving nurse-doctor communication would improve care. All too often, says Pike, physicians develop **treatment plans** in isolation from nursing treatment plans. Doctors may conduct **rounds** by themselves, without nurses' input. Though physicians talk about cases with individual nurses, groups of doctors do not regularly meet with groups of nurses to discuss problems or successes in their respective routines. "So the end result," Pike says, "is physician- and nursing-**care plans** that never even see each other. A lot of physicians aren't even aware that there is such a thing as a nursing-care plan."

Pike and the physicians she recruited have changed all that. Doctors and nurses go on rounds together every morning. That way nurses can alert physicians to what a patient will be doing on that particular day, Pike explains: "We tell them, for example, this is going to be a high-activity day for the patient. He'll be starting to walk today—maybe 250 feet down the hall. This may mean he'll need more pain medication. Or we'll know the patient is going home that day and we'll explain the kind of nursing concerns we have."

One of the most important issues they grapple with is how the physicians can recognize the role of nurses in deciding when and how to terminate "heroic treatment"—that is, life support systems and **resuscitation** of dying patients. When patients, doctors, families, and nurses decide that a patient's condition is **terminal** and that heroic measures only **prolong** suffering, physicians generally write a do not resuscitate (**DNR**) order. But nurses on Seven North, like nurses all over the country, have come to realize that there are many invisible conflicts that such an order can't solve.

"If you have a DNR order, sometimes people think it just means we don't try to resuscitate a patient who has **cardiac arrest,** but a DNR order involves many other things," Pike says. Do nurses continue with **antibiotics?** Do nurses put a tube down a dying patient's nose to draw fluid from the lung? "I remember when I drew blood on a patient who was very old and frail. There was a DNR order, but there I was, **probing** around these very frail veins for blood. The skin was just"—Pike pauses, shudders at the memory, and gropes for the right word—"it was just like thin antique parchment. I tried to make the needle very, very fine to be gentle. But you felt you were torturing her."

Because many physicians have not been trained to value nurses' experience and insight, when nurses see treatment as torture they often have no recourse other than what Pike calls "moral outrage." On her unit, nurses have tried to turn that outrage into lessons that can benefit all medical personnel and, more importantly, the patients they care for. In the process, she says, the two professions also learn to understand and empathize with each other. Pike recounts the story of a physician who had trouble going into a dying patient's room. He explained that the man reminded him of his father: "Suddenly, we all saw this physician from a very different perspective."

The need for a powerful nursing voice has never been greater. In a PBS special on the nation's health-care crisis, Walter Cronkite stated the problem succinctly. Our health-care system, he said, is neither healthy nor caring, nor even a system. Recognition of nurses' expertise and importance is critical to changing that.

Real health care, of course, involves far more than paying physicians to intervene when disease is well established or financing dazzling research into potential "cures." It involves education in **disease prevention** and **health maintenance** from childhood through old age, as well as providing skilled nursing care in hospitals when patients are **acutely** ill. A truly humane system would not push **futile** treatment on patients with terminal diseases, but would permit them to die in comfort and with dignity. A genuinely economical health-care system would finance a cohesive network of **long-term care** to be provided outside of big hospitals in the home and the community.

Nursing is already injecting these considerations into our conception of medical care, but imagine how rapidly these efforts would advance if we created a health-care system that valued care as much as cure. Working in collaboration with physicians, nurse practitioners would manage patient care, with quality—not simply cost containment—as the watchword. They would identify those at risk for particular illnesses and recommend either immediate treatment or long-term monitoring of a patient's condition. In **health-care clinics,** physicians' **private practices,** and **health-maintenance organizations,** nurses would routinely scan patients' records to make sure that recommended follow-up care was actually administered. Because quality care goes beyond regular office encounters, nurses would keep in touch with patients to schedule **follow-up treatment** and address any fears and anxieties patients may have about returning to the doctor, thus **minimizing** the chance that a minor **complaint** will **escalate** into a **catastrophic** illness.

Instead of seeing physicians as the only ones in charge of **acute care,** hospitals would emphasize the collaborative nature of treatment. Nurses, hospitals could explain, are the ones who have the time to clarify doctors' advice, explore the ramifications and **side effects** of treatments and high-tech chemical and surgical measures, teach patients how to cope with a reduced level of functioning, describe what will happen after **discharge,** discuss in-home care, and deal with the termination of life-support systems.

Nurses, moreover, would officially be able to ask hard questions: Does an 85-year-old man really need **coronary bypass surgery?** Is it fair to keep a patient on a **ventilator,** or would it be more humane to let her die with dignity? Could a patient be better cared for at home, and how could family and friends effectively provide that care? Most importantly, the benefits of genuine nurse-doctor collaboration would become a standard lesson in a physician's education.

All of these changes and many more, of course, would be reflected and reinforced in the political solutions to our health-care crisis. Nurses with advanced education would be allowed to **prescribe medication** and be paid accordingly for the additional care they'd provide. Americans would be able to choose **practitioners, nurse midwives,** clinical nurse specialists, **nurse anesthetists,** and **public-health nurses.**

Reforming our medical system in ways that would give nurses broader roles and greater financial rewards will indeed cost money, but these costs can be offset by limiting physicians' fees, curtailing unnecessary medical procedures, and eliminating the extraordinary waste of a private-insurance-based health-care system in which 23 percent of funds are spent on administration of

1,500 different insurance plans. Ultimately, when expert nurses like Betsy Gemmell and Janet Craig are allowed to build trust with patients, teach people to care for sick loved ones, and reassure patients or relatives deciding to forgo extraordinary treatments, they are saving lives and anguish, and money as well.

To create this new health-care system, nurses need to be far less humble and far more assertive in promoting their profession and its achievements. They also need advocates and allies—among patients, families, politicians, businesspeople, and journalists—who understand that high-quality health care is dependent not only on technology, fancy surgery, and the promise of cure, but also on the efforts of hundreds of thousands of women and men who provide the care without which the cure would be impossible.

Comprehension and Discussion Questions

These discussion questions ask you to locate important information in the article, as well as analyze carefully and think critically about information in the reading. Use 10–15 new words from the reading to answer the questions. In small groups, discuss your answers to these questions.

1. Following the title of this article, Gordon claims that "an expanded role for nurses would bring healthy results to our medical system" (page 18). What does this say about the author's point of view or perspective about nursing? What words does she use to reflect her point of view? Why does the author use *would bring* instead of *brings* in the subtitle?
2. Gordon writes that "the relationship between caring and curing. . . [is] at the heart of nursing" (page 18). Explain what Gordon means.
3. List at least five responsibilities of a nurse.
4. What is "primary nursing" (page 19)? How does it differ from regular nursing? What are the benefits of primary nursing?
5. Why is trust so important in the relationship between a patient and nurse?
6. What is collaborative care between doctors and nurses? Describe how collaborative care differs from traditional care. What are the benefits of collaborative care?
7. What is a DNR order? What are some of the "many invisible conflicts that such an order can't solve" (page 20)?
8. On page 21, Gordon sets up a hypothetical condition about health care reform: "if we created a health care system that valued care as much as cure." How would the responsibilities of nurses change if this were true? List six responsibilities. Are these changes likely to occur, do you think? Why or why not?
9. What do nurses need to do to implement these reforms, according to the author? Do you think this will be difficult for nurses to do? Why or why not?
10. Now that you have read the article and answered the questions, what do you think Gordon's purpose was in writing the article? Was the author effective in accomplishing her purpose? Why or why not?

Vocabulary Strategies and Skills

In nursing there are many specialized terms you will need to learn. Many colleges and universities offer a course in medical terminology that you should take before you begin your nursing program. That way, you can avoid having to learn medical terminology at the same time you are learning nursing content.

The work in this unit cannot possibly replace a medical terminology course, but it will introduce you to strategies and skills that will help you learn new vocabulary more easily.

In addition to specialized vocabulary, you are introduced to vocabulary from a variety of other fields, such as psychology, sociology, economics, ethics, and cultural studies, all reflecting the many influences on nursing.

Using Context Clues

One way to learn some new words is to understand as much as you can from the context surrounding the word. Sometimes there is a clue in the context that will help you understand its meaning. If you can figure out the meaning of a word from its context, you avoid having to interrupt your reading to look up the definition in a dictionary. This saves time and allows you to stay focused on the reading. Your understanding of the word will fit the context. When you use a dictionary, you still have to select the correct definition. Words often have several meanings, and it is not always obvious which meaning or definition is the most appropriate one unless you look at the context.

A few types of clues that the context of a word can provide are words with a similar meaning; words used in contrast; definitions of words, both direct and indirect; and the general context.

The examples on pages 25–29 illustrate each type of clue.

Words with a Similar Meaning

1. Look for words that are similar in meaning to the word you don't know. To be descriptive as well as persuasive, writers often use several words together that are similar in meaning.

   Example

   Nurses have the time to explain the **ramifications** and *side effects* of treatments.

   Ramifications means "results or effects of something you do." It is similar in meaning to *side effects.*

2. Look for **synonyms.** Writers sometimes use synonyms to avoid repeating the same word; they replace one word with another word to avoid repetition.

   Example

   Water may simply be poured over the **corpse** . . . the *body* is wrapped in one or two white cotton shrouds and placed in a plain wooden coffin.

   Corpse and *body* are synonyms; they are used interchangeably in the reading.

3. Look for **connecting words and phrases** that indicate a similarity in meaning. Writers sometimes use certain words and phrases to connect ideas that are similar, such as: *likewise, similarly, in the same way, by the same token, part of,* etc.

   Example

   Registered nurses are discontented for many reasons. . . . The **discontent** *is part of* a broader *malaise* that also affects physicians and others who work in hospitals.

   The phrase *is part of* connects **discontent** with its synonym, *malaise.* The discontent that nurses are feeling is part of a broader discontent, which physicians and others are feeling, too. To avoid repeating the word **discontent,** a synonym is used instead.

Words Used in Contrast

1. Look for words that are opposite in meaning to the word you don't know. Writers sometimes develop an idea in opposition or in contrast to another.

   Example

   The patient is lying in a state somewhere *between consciousness* and **coma.**

   Coma is a "state of unconsciousness from which a person cannot be awakened by external stimuli." *Consciousness* and **coma** are presented as two opposite ends of a continuum; the word *between* helps to set up this contrast.

2. Look for **antonyms.**

   Example

   Learning about West Africa's cultural beliefs allowed the instructor to teach psychiatric nursing in a way that **integrated,** *rather than dismantled,* the students' cultural beliefs.

   Integrate means to combine two or more things in order to make an effective system; *dismantle* means to take something apart. The phrase *rather than* sets up these two words in opposition to each other.

3. Look for the word *not,* which signals a contrast.

   Example

   Although clinicians are prohibited from taking positive action to bring about death, they are also not to maintain any treatments that are *not* **curative** *but only prolong the dying process.*

   Use of the word *not* immediately before the word **curative,** followed by *but only prolong the dying process* suggests that curative means the opposite of something that prolongs the process of dying. Indeed, curative refers to something that can make a patient healthy again.

4. Look for **connecting words and phrases** that indicate a contrast in meaning. Writers sometimes use certain words and phrases to show a relationship of contrast or opposition, such as: *but, although, whereas, however, on the other hand, on the contrary, in contrast, nevertheless,* and *despite,* etc.

   Example

   The wife supports the family by working in a **menial** job *while* the husband attempts to find *professional* employment.

   The connecting word *while* indicates a relationship of contrast between **menial** job and *professional* employment. Menial is the opposite of professional.

5. Look for **adverbs** with a negative meaning, such as *never, rarely, only, barely, merely,* and *hardly.*

   Example

   The illness is *rarely,* if ever, **curable.**

   Use of the word *rarely* suggests a negative outcome of an illness. **Curable** means an illness that can be stopped, so an illness that is rarely curable is one that most likely cannot be stopped.

6. Look for words with negative **prefixes,** such as: *un-, in-, im-, il-, ir-, non-, a-,* and *dis-*.

   Example

   For young refugees, the pressure to conform simultaneously to American and Vietnamese cultures—which are in many ways **incompatible**—is a major source of strain.

   The prefix *in-* indicates a negative meaning. American and Vietnamese cultures are different cultures. Although difference is not necessarily negative, those differences that are **incompatible** are a major source of strain for younger refugees, who feel the pressure from two different directions. From the context, you can figure out that incompatible differences refers to cultural differences that are too great to overcome.

Definitions of Words

Look for definitions of words in the context. Writers often include definitions of important words that may be unfamiliar to their readers. This is especially the case when the writer is not addressing experts on a topic, but the general public. These definitions can be either direct or indirect.

Direct Definitions

1. Look for a formal definition from a dictionary or other official source, such as a textbook. Formal definitions are often set off by quotation marks, if they have been copied from an outside source, followed by a citation of the source. Definitions are also sometimes introduced by verbs, such as *states* followed by *that* and a noun clause.

   Example

   The principle of **autonomy** underlying informed consent *states that* if patients are sufficiently knowledgeable about their condition and treatment options, are free from constraint and are mentally competent, then they have the right and responsibility to make choices and to exercise informed consent.

   The definition of **autonomy** is provided immediately after the words *states that.*

2. Look for a definition or synonym set off by commas and the word *or.*

   Example

   Another ethical principle undergirding consent is **veracity** *or* truth-telling on the part of the health care provider.

   Veracity and *truth-telling* are synonyms, connected by the word *or.*

3. Look for a definition set off by commas or other forms of **punctuation,** such as **commas, parentheses,** or **dashes**.

   Example: Commas

   In such an instance, autonomy conflicts with **beneficence,** *the mandate of physicians to act for the good of the patient.*

   The definition of **beneficence** is: *the mandate of physicians to act for the good of the patient.* The definition is set off from *beneficence* by a comma.

   Example: Parentheses

   Realizing that the patient is having an **anaphylactic reaction** *(her airway is swelling and closing),* the nurse immediately turns a small spigot on the IV tubing to shut off the drip.

   The definition "*airway is swelling and closing*" is provided in parentheses immediately after the term: **anaphylactic reaction.**

   Example: Dashes

   Then the nurse checks her **vital signs**—*temperature, blood pressure, heart and respiratory rate*—and examines the area around the point of entry of her intravenous tube.

   The definition *temperature, blood pressure, heart and respiratory rate* is provided between dashes immediately after the term: **vital signs.**

Indirect Definitions

1. Look for examples that help define a word.

   Example

   The herbal mixture was placed in all **orifices** of the victim, *i.e., nose, mouth, rectum,* and even *ears and eyes* because spirits are thought to enter the individual via the body openings.

   Some examples are set off by abbreviations, such as e.g. or i.e. In this instance, examples of **orifices** are set off by *i.e.* By looking at the examples: *nose, mouth, rectum, ears, and eyes,* you can figure out that **orifices** refers to openings in the body.

2. Look for connecting words and phrases that are used to introduce examples and details, such as: *for example, for instance, such as,* and *including.*

   Example

   Women are not permitted to follow a funeral procession in order to avoid ritual **lamentation,** *such as* striking one's face or tearing at one's hair, or other open displays of emotion.

   The phrase *such as,* set off by a comma, introduces two examples of **lamentation:** striking one's face or tearing at one's hair, and then as the third example, provides a partial definition of the word: open display of emotion. From the examples, you can figure out that lamentation is an open display of extreme grief or sadness.

General Context

1. Sometimes there is not a specific clue, but by reading the sentence or paragraph in which the word occurs, you can make an educated guess about what it means.

   Example

   Wires connect him to a series of **monitors** that provide second-by-second displays of his heart and respiratory rhythms.

   From the context, you can figure out that a monitor is a piece of equipment that provides second-by-second displays of heart and respiratory rhythms.

2. **Pronouns** usually replace nouns or noun phrases. Sometimes they can replace verb phrases. They can even replace clauses or sentences. Sometimes by understanding what pronouns are referring to, you can figure out the overall meaning of an unfamiliar word.

   Example

   Craig concentrates on reducing her patient's anxiety about both her condition and the high-tech treatment she is receiving. She sees that *the girl is becoming very* **agitated** and that *this* might **aggravate** her condition. So she tries to calm and reassure her, explaining what the doctors and nurses are doing and why.

   This replaces the clause the girl is becoming very agitated. Since, *becoming agitated* is not good, **aggravate** must have a negative meaning; indeed, it means "to worsen."

General versus Specialized Definitions

Some words used in the field of nursing or medicine have both general and specialized meanings. A regular dictionary may have the specialized definitions of commonly used medical terms, but many specialized words can only be found in a medical dictionary.

For example, *bipolar* is a word with both general and specialized meanings. It is used in Reading 4.1 (see page 129).

Activity: Understanding General versus Specialized Definitions

Look up the work *bipolar* in a college English dictionary, and write both the general and specialized definitions:

1. *General* definition of *bipolar:* ________________________________
2. *Specialized* definition of *bipolar:* ________________________________
3. Look at the context of this word in the reading on page 129. Is the word meant in the general or specialized sense? ____________________
4. Often the general meaning gives students a clue to the specialized meaning. What is similar about the two definitions of *bipolar*?

   ____

Activity: More General versus Specialized Definitions

The words below are commonly used in nursing, but they are also commonly used in their more general sense, as well. Look up these words in both a college English dictionary and a medical English dictionary, and discuss the differences and similarities between the definitions given. If there is more than one definition in the college English dictionary, choose the first one.

1. monitor (n.)
2. dressing (n.)
3. discharge (n.)
4. evacuation (n.)
5. prescribe (v.)
6. administer (v.)
7. present (v.)
8. terminal (adj.)
9. sterile (adj.)
10. compliant (adj.)

Parts of Speech

Many words can be changed into different parts of speech, for example, from a noun to a verb or from a verb to an adjective. When you look up a word in a dictionary, you may not find all its parts of speech.

For example, *somatize* and *somatization* are both used in Reading 4.1 (see page 132). *Somatize* is a verb; *somatization* is a noun.

Look up both words in a medical English dictionary and write their definitions:

somatize (v.): ____

somatization (n.): ____

Some dictionaries include only *somatization.* If *somatize* is not listed in your dictionary, look at the definition of *somatization* and figure out the definition of the verb from the noun.

Three activities on the parts of speech follow on pages 31–32.

Parts of Speech 1

These nouns are from Reading 1.2. Look up any words you do not know in a medical English dictionary and write the definition. Then, change the nouns into verbs and/or adjectives.

Nouns	Verbs	Adjectives
1. monitor	__________	__________
2. operation	__________	__________
3. hospitalization	__________	__________
4. dressing	__________	__________
5. treatment	__________	__________
6. resuscitation	__________	__________
7. prevention	__________	__________
8. maintenance	__________	__________
9. complaint	__________	__________
10. discharge	__________	__________
11. ventilator	__________	__________
12. medication	__________	__________

Parts of Speech 2

These verbs are from Reading 1.2. Look up any words you do not know in a medical English dictionary and write the definition. Then, change the words into nouns and/or adjectives.

Verbs	Nouns	Adjectives
1. implant	__________	__________
2. assess	__________	__________
3. prolong	__________	__________
4. probe	__________	__________
5. minimize	__________	__________
6. prescribe	__________	__________

Parts of Speech 3

These adjectives are from Reading 1.2. Look up any words you do not know in a medical English dictionary and write the definition. Then, change the adjectives into nouns and verbs.

Adjectives	Nouns	Verbs
1. pediatric	__________	__________
2. respiratory	__________	__________
3. sedated	__________	__________
4. diagnostic	__________	__________
5. metastatic	__________	__________
6. circulatory	__________	__________
7. recurring	__________	__________
8. terminal	__________	__________

Checking Definitions

When you look up a word in a dictionary, check the definition you select using the original context of the word. Reread the sentence or paragraph in which the word occurred, and substitute the definition, instead of the original word. Does the sentence make sense?

For example, look at the original context of the word *bipolar* on p. 129. Substitute the general definition of *bipolar* into the original sentence. If necessary, make minor adjustments so that the grammar and meaning of the sentence do not change.

<u>Original</u>
Media reports and academic research reveal—and often overemphasize—the *bipolar* adaptation of Vietnamese youth.

<u>With substitution of definition</u>
Media reports and academic research reveal—and often overemphasize—the adaptation of Vietnamese youth *that consists of two opposite trends.*

Online Resources

The following online dictionary may be a helpful resource:

www.online-medical-dictionary.org/

One website offers links to information and exercises on prefixes, suffixes, roots, and pronunciation:

http://ec.hku.hk/mt/

Another website provides a list of both technical and popular medical terms:

http://users.ugent.be/~rvdstich/eugloss/EN/lijst.html

Activity: Vocabulary Development

Words that have been selected for vocabulary study for Reading 1.2 are all specialized medical/nursing terms. (In this reading, and in all subsequent readings, selected vocabulary words are in bold type.) Create your own dictionary of new words using a spiral notebook. Include only those words that you do not know.

1. Write the word, part of speech, and the original context of the word. For the context, write out the phrase, clause, or complete sentence the word appears in, just enough so you can see the word in its original context. For example, for the first word in bold type, **pediatric,** notice that it describes the noun *unit* and therefore is an adjective. For the context, write the introductory phrase and underline the selected word: in the pediatric intensive care unit at UCSF Medical Center.
2. Try to figure out the meaning of the word, using context clues if available.
3. Use a medical English dictionary to look up the words you do not know; a general dictionary will not necessarily give you the specialized definition of how words are used in nursing or medicine. Write a brief definition of the words you do not know.

Writing about Nursing: Understanding and Synthesizing Information

Now that you have read and discussed about nursing as a profession, choose one of the following topics and write an essay of two or three pages. These topics require you to understand and synthesize information from the readings and from your own personal experience.

1. What is nursing? Write a brief essay about nursing as a profession. Include a definition of nursing and discuss the responsibilities, challenges, and rewards of nursing with specific examples of each.
2. Why do you want to be a nurse? What characteristics of the profession attract you to it? What kind of work do you want to do as a nurse, in terms of specialty and setting? Write a brief essay that addresses these issues.
3. Write a brief essay that compares and contrasts the profession of nursing in your native country and in the United States. Provide specific examples of differences. What are some of the reasons for these differences? Would you prefer to be a nurse in the United States or in your native country? Explain your answer.

UNIT

2

Thinking Critically about Nursing

The **content-based objectives** include learning about

- Factors contributing to the nursing shortage
- Ways in which changes in the health care system have affected nurses, the profession of nursing, and patient care

The **skill-based objectives** include

- Critical reading skills
  - making inferences
  - analyzing and synthesizing information
  - applying and evaluating information
- Critical-thinking skills
  - evaluating sources of information
  - understanding the author's perspective and purpose for writing and his or her influence on the content and tone
- Reading and interpreting information in figures

At the end of the unit, you will reflect on your understanding of the nursing shortage and its effect on the profession of nursing.

Activating Prior Knowledge about a Topic

This unit focuses on critical reading skills and understanding figures, while exploring contemporary issues in nursing. Some of the issues you will explore are: the nursing shortage and how the role of nursing has evolved as a result of changes in the health care system.

Think about and answer these questions.

1. Do you and/or your family have health insurance? If not, why? If so, have you been satisfied with the coverage? Why or why not?
2. Has a member of your family been hospitalized within the last five years? What was the quality of nursing care that he or she received? Provide specific examples.
3. Do you know anyone who has worked as a nurse for the past five years? If so, ask her or him if and how working conditions have changed. Also, ask what the greatest concerns are about working as a nurse today.

Critical Reading Skills

When you read to simply understand and learn the information contained in a reading, that level of understanding is called comprehension. While comprehension is essential for all kinds of reading, much more is involved in critical reading. **Critical reading** is the ability to engage in higher-order thinking, such as making inferences, analyzing and synthesizing information, and applying and evaluating information. For example, you may need to **infer** something that was not stated directly or form your own conclusion about information given in the text. You might need to **analyze** the text or take apart the ideas and look at them one by one in order to better understand them. Or, you may need to **synthesize** or put together information from several different sources by looking for patterns in the information (such as similarities or differences) and then integrating the information into a new way of presenting or understanding it. You might need to **apply** information from one kind of situation to another or **evaluate** the accuracy of information or its usefulness for a particular situation. These are higher-order thinking/critical reading skills.

Critical Thinking in Nursing

The job of a nurse requires considerable critical thinking. As defined in Kozier et al.'s (2004a) *Fundamentals of Nursing*, it is "the intellectually disciplined process of actively and skillfully conceptualizing, applying, analyzing, synthesizing, and/or evaluating information gathered from, or generated by, observation, experience, reflection, reasoning, or communication, as a guide to belief and action" (p. 245).

In nursing, critical thinking is most often associated with the nursing process of assessing, diagnosing, planning, implementing, and evaluating. For example, when you assess the physical and psychosocial needs of a client (analyze and synthesize), you then need to determine an appropriate nursing diagnosis (infer), plan and implement an appropriate intervention (apply), and evaluate the effectiveness of the intervention (evaluate).

In your nursing studies, it is important to be able to read critically, to understand a reading within its broader context, and to recognize the influences of culture and context on the reading and its meaning. In addition, research-based writing requires you to use multiple outside sources to explore a particular topic, for which analysis, synthesis, and evaluation are especially important skills.

Evaluation is also used in the sense of critiquing or challenging information in a reading. For example, it involves recognizing an author's bias in the selection, presentation, and analysis of information and in a research study, recognizing flaws in the design of the study or in the analysis of data. (See pages 100–1 in Unit 3 on writing a critique.) It may also involve presenting your own ideas and opinions with respect to a particular issue.

In research-based writing, you need to have a critical eye regarding your sources of information, especially if they are from the Internet. You must evaluate their credibility (College of St. Catherine Libraries, 2005) (see pages 87–88 in Unit 3 on evaluating information from websites) just as you should evaluate the credentials and the purpose of the author to determine the credibility of the information itself.

Some of the questions you should ask are:

- Who are the authors?
- What are their credentials?
- Do they have expertise in the area they are writing about?
- Who published the article? Is the publisher reputable, or did the author self-publish either in print or on the Internet? If on the Internet, was it through an individual website or a website associated with a university, professional organization, government agency, company, or special interest group?
- When was the article published? Is the information outdated? Or is it still relevant?
- If the article was based on research, who funded the research? Was there a possible conflict of interest between the purpose of the study and the source of funding?
- Do the authors have a particular perspective or bias in their approach to the topic? If so, did they make their perspective clear or is it hidden?

Activity: Evaluating Sources of Information

This unit has three readings. Preview them for information about the authors, their credentials and professional background, the magazine or journal the reading was published in (the source), and the intended audience. For each reading, answer the questions.

1. Who are the authors?

   R2.1 ______________________________

   R2.2 ______________________________

   R2.3 ______________________________

2. What are their credentials? Are they credible sources of information about nursing? Why or why not? How might their professional background influence their perspective about the nursing crisis in the United States?

   R2.1 ______________________________

   R2.2 ______________________________

   R2.3 ______________________________

3. When were these articles originally published? Do you think any of these articles are out-of-date? Why or why not?

   R2.1 ____

   R2.2 ____

   R2.3 ____

4. In what journals or magazines were these articles originally published? What kind of journals or magazines are they? (Check your library or the Internet for more information about them.)

   R2.1 ____

   R2.2 ____

   R2.3 ____

5. Who do you think was the author's intended audience?

   R2.1 ____

   R2.2 ____

   R2.3 ____

Understanding Different Perspectives

The three readings in this unit relate in some way to contemporary issues in nursing, but the authors' perspectives and purposes for writing are not the same, and neither are the content and tone. Determining how the articles differ and why they differ is part of developing a critical awareness when you read.

Reading 2.1 is an excerpt from the article "The Evolution of a Crisis: Nursing in America," which discusses various factors contributing to the current nursing crisis. Reading 2.2, "Nurse, Interrupted," exposes ways in which hospital restructuring and the downsizing of nursing have affected not only the quality of patient care, but also the physical and psychological well-being of nurses. Reading 2.3, "Nursing in the Crossfire," provides yet another perspective on the current nursing shortage. Reading 2.3 covers many of the same topics as the other two readings: current nursing shortage, dissatisfaction among nurses, and legislative initiatives, but the nature of the supporting data and the tone of the article are quite different.

Answer the comprehension and discussion questions, and consider the authors' perspectives, the contents of the readings, and their tone.

Reading 2.1

The Evolution of a Crisis: Nursing in America

Bobbi Kimball, MBA, RN, received her BSN from the University of Florida and an MBA from the University of San Francisco. Bobbi is a health care management consultant with 25 years of experience designing and implementing innovative change.

Edward O'Neil, PhD, is a professor of Family and Community Medicine and Dental Public Health at the University of California at San Francisco, where he also serves as director of the Center for the Health Professions.

Authors' Note: The authors wish to thank the Robert Wood Johnson Foundation, California HealthCare Foundation, and California Endowment for their support of this work. The views expressed are those of the authors.

A recent study by the American Hospital Association found that "hospitals find themselves facing both immediate and long-term shortages of personnel" (American Hospital Association, 2001, p. 3). These were not limited to nurses, but included all types of allied health personnel and entry-level clerical and custodial staff as well. A more recent study by the Center for the Health Professions points to a similar shortage in nursing that runs the gamut of nursing employment across sectors of the health system and regions of California (Coffman, Spetz, Seago, Rosenoff, & O'Neil, 2001). Indeed, a number of studies from a wide variety of professional and industry associations have now tagged the nursing shortage as the current crisis in health care.

This reality is being driven by a **confluence** of powerful forces, many of which reach beyond health care. The most significant force is the aging of the U.S. population.

Figure 1 shows the trends in five-year age **cohorts** in the year 2010 for California. If anything, California is younger than the rest of the nation so the trends for the aging population are likely to be more severe elsewhere. There are three things that the graph reveals in dramatic detail. First, the population in general is aging, and this means that health care workers, all health care workers, are aging along with the general population. The average age of registered nurses (RNs) in California is 49, but this is no more alarming than other trends in other professions. The fact of the matter is that the U.S. workforce is aging and older people will be doing more of the work than in the past. For professions where the entry age has grown older, such as nursing and other allied professions, or in which the work is physically demanding and may not be able to be done by those of a certain age, the workforce will be even more constrained. Nursing faces an uncertain future in this regard.

The second dimension revealed by this graph is the size of the aging cohorts that represent the **baby boom.** As this generation of more than 76 million ages past 60, they can be expected to begin to consume more health care and utilize more health services. If in fact an aging population translates into a growth in demand for health service, then it will inevitably create a demand for more health workers. We have few models of possible change in the demand for service, but historically, as people age they have more and more complex disease and disability. This pattern seems unlikely to change in the future, but there are scenarios offered that have a more self-reliant consumer, one more focused on maintaining health into older years. Which pattern of consumer use of the health care system arrives as the first Boomers hit the Medicare program in 2011 remains to be seen.

Figure 1 California Total Population 2010 by 5-Year Cohorts in Millions

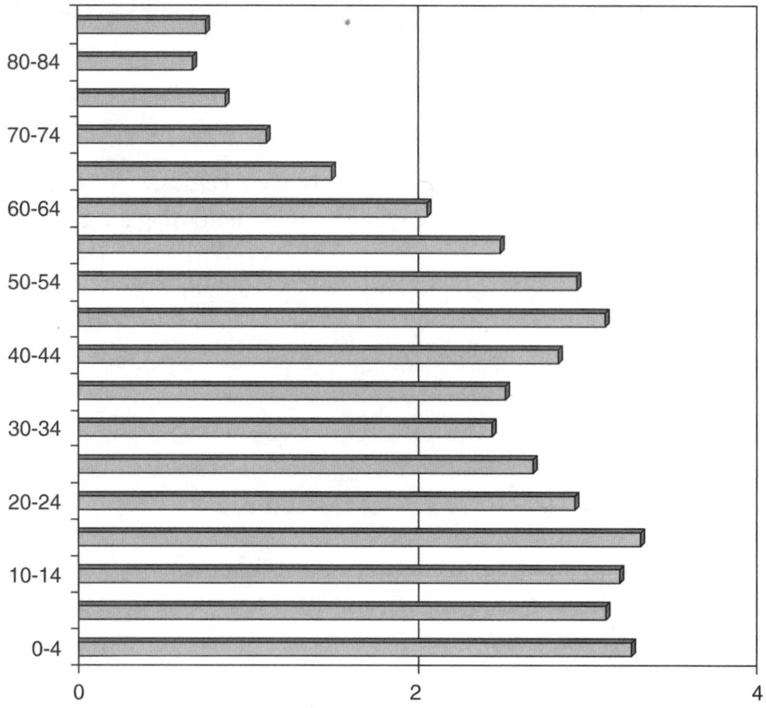

Source: California Department of Finance.

The final demographic reality of this chart is the **demise** of the size of the cohorts that immediately follow the Boomers. The graph reveals a gap that will be hard to overcome. Workers in this age group are competitively sought after and industry outside of the health sector is already aggressively positioning itself for what it perceives as the **impending war for talent.** What they mean by this is that success in the future will not be merely filling the work rolls. Success in a rapidly changing technological environment and in an age of a **shrinking** entry cohort will mean the ability to attract and retain workers that have the very best technological and interpersonal skills. The reality is that if an employer is having difficulty attracting such workers today, the challenge will grow dramatically in the future.

In addition to issues related to the age distribution of society is the movement from a mainstream Caucasian majority culture to a multicultural reality that blends a rich and very diverse set of ethnic and cultural minorities into the overall U.S. population. This past year [2000], California joined Hawaii and New Mexico as a **non-majority** state for the entire population, but if one looks at the population younger than 15, the majority returns but as a Latino majority. This reality will be uneven across the United States, but as institutions struggle to cope with the changes driven by age, they will of necessity do so in a cultural environment that is changing as well.

The second large trend affecting the nursing crisis is the continued **stress** of the health care delivery organization. For most of the post–World War II period, hospitals, clinics, health plans, and colleges and schools for training and educating professionals lived under the regime of a growing industry (from 5 percent of the **gross domestic product** in 1960 to 14 percent in [2001]). There was little external **accountability** or **mandates** for such a system. Run as a **cost plus reimbursed enterprise** for so many years, all of health care has become used to its particular way of organizing and providing care services. Although much good has been done under such an operation, by the mid-1990s, the purchasers began to be concerned about overall cost and effectiveness of the system.

For the past decade or so [1991–2001], unevenly across the country, the "system" of care has moved to become more accountable for cost and outcomes. This adjustment has and will continue to create enormous stress and dislocation in the system. This stress has trickled down into the workplace in many different forms: perceived shortness of physician exam time, reduction in middle managers in hospitals, more acute and thereby stressful patient care loads, more competition between and among professional groups, and more demanding environments and fewer and tighter resources in general.

This has made health care employment less fulfilling, more contentious, and more filled with stress than ever before. Hospitals have been the **epicenter** of much of this stress, and it has translated into work environments for nurses that are more demanding, less fulfilling, and more stressful. As this environment seems to have become **intractable** in some places, it has left many nurses **disillusioned** with their ability to provide competent and professional care. This dissatisfaction has led to both difficulty in retaining nurses and recruiting new nurses in many settings. Though unmeasured, such widespread dissatisfaction with professional practice must have a negative impact on the long-term ability to attract young people into the nursing profession.

The third development that is driving the unfolding nursing crisis is one of values. Although many values issues are relevant to the overall trend, there are two significant **shifts** that are particularly relevant driving most of the action. First is the value women place on nursing as a career. Undoubtedly, the profession has benefited historically from the limited number of legitimate options for professional careers for women. Nursing and teaching drew large numbers to the calling of their work but also provided one of the few **outlets** for women desiring to serve or needing to work. This reality has obviously changed, and women desiring entry into a health profession find few of the barriers that their mothers or grandmothers faced. Such choices for women cannot be regretted and little can be done about it. However, a couple of interesting questions are: Why, even with the choice available, have women left nursing? and Why, given new opportunities, have men not entered in numbers significant enough to make a major difference in overall numbers?

The other relevant value shift is around generational values and work. The values of Generation X, the generation that is most sought after these days for education and employment, differ dramatically from those that are most **viably** represented by the hospital and much of nursing (Tulgan, 2000). These sets of values are presented in Table 1. Clearly, a part of what is creating the nursing crisis is a general disconnect between the **aspirations** of this generation and the ways in which nursing practice is perceived.

The final trend is the general shift in the nature of work. Beginning in the late 1980s and quickening throughout the decade of the '90s, the very nature and organization of work in the United States and truly around the globe has changed. These changes represent a broad switch from industrial forms of productivity to a more **service-oriented undertaking.** This revolution was already afoot in the United States in the early 1960s (Miles, 1976) but moved into a much more extensive undertaking by the deeper **penetration** of information and communications technology into the economy and society in general (Evans & Wurster, 2000). These changes have occurred within the landscape of an even more fundamental pattern of work organization and firm ownership.

These changes have led to a more varied workplace with the rise of new **entrepreneurial** opportunities for individuals where once little was available except employment in large corporate settings (Handy, 1994). As the nature of employment and institutional life changes, pushed by the drive of information technology, health care has generally been left behind. This need not happen. Some settings and some professional practices in health care are marked by flexibility and the use

Table 1 Comparison of Generation X Values and Hospital Image

Generation X Desires	Hospital Image
Service oriented	On strike, laid-off, Angels of Mercy
Anti-institutional	Work in large, cold, unresponsive institutions
Not hierarchical	
Flexible, change welcoming	Work is stressful, highly structured, and unfun
Diversity	
Technology	Lack the high-tech access associated with medicine
New skills	Tied to a professional career, not open to change
Community of work	

Source: Coffman, Spetz, Seago, Rosenoff, and O'Neil (2001).

of current technology across a broad **spectrum.** Other settings and professions, however, have not been involved in such a revolution. Ultimately, the challenge will be for institutions of health care to be more competitive with a broader U.S. work environment that is faster, **flatter,** and more flexible than what most health care settings offer. The confluence of these major developments of demography, a changing health care system, changing social values, and **alteration** in the nature of work in general create the overwhelming nature of the nursing crisis today. The size and complexity of these changes mean that responses to nursing shortages in the past will be inadequate to the task today.

References

American Hospital Association. (2001). *Workforce supply for hospitals and health systems issues and recommendations.* Chicago: AHA.

California Department of Finance. *Profile of aging.*

Coffman, J., Spetz, J., Seago, J. A., Rosenoff, E., & O'Neil, E. (2001). *Nursing in California: A workforce crisis.* San Francisco: Center for the Health Professions.

Evans, P., & Wurster, T. (2000). *Blown to bits.* Boston: Harvard Business School Press.

Handy, C. (1994). *The age of paradox.* Boston: Harvard Business School Press.

Miles, R. E. (1976). *Awakening from the American dream: The social and political limits to growth.* New York: Universe Books.

Tulgan, B. (2000). *Managing Generation X.* New York: Norton.

Activity: Vocabulary Development

Reading 2.1 contains many socio-economic terms that are used to describe the current crisis in nursing. Add the words you do not know to your dictionary, following the guidelines on page 33. Use a college-level English dictionary to look up words you do not know. Use 10–15 new words in answering the discussion questions.

Comprehension and Discussion Questions

These questions ask you to locate important information in Reading 2.1, as well as analyze carefully and think critically about information in the reading. In small groups, discuss your answers to these questions.

1. What are three demographic factors, reflected in Figure 1 (page 42), that have led to a short- and long-term nursing shortage?
2. Why do you think the "movement from a mainstream Caucasian majority culture to a multicultural reality that blends a rich and very diverse set of ethnic and cultural minorities into the overall U.S. population" (page 42) is significant in a discussion of the current nursing crisis?
3. What are some of the ways in which the changes in the health care system "to become more accountable for cost and outcomes" (page 43) have affected the workplace?
4. How have these changes in the workplace affected nurses and efforts to recruit and retain nurses?
5. How has the attitude of women toward a career in nursing changed over the years? What are the reasons given for this change in attitude? What do you think are some ways that women today could become more interested in a career in nursing?
6. How are the values of Generation X, listed in Table 1 (page 44), different from the values associated with the nursing profession and hospital employment? What do you think are some ways that the nursing profession and hospital administrators could interest members of Generation X in a career in nursing?
7. How has the nature of work changed since the 1990s? How have these changes affected nursing?

Reading 2.2

Nurse, Interrupted

Suzanne Gordon is an author and journalist from Boston. She is the author or co-author of ten books on nursing and health care. Gordon is co-editor of the Cornell University Press series on the Culture and Politics of Health Care Work. She is also Assistant Adjunct Professor at the University of California–San Francisco's School of Nursing.

It's May 13, the day after Florence Nightingale's birthday, and as part of the annual celebration of Nurses' Week—established in part to commemorate Nightingale's role in the development of professional nursing—members of the Massachusetts Nurses Association have asked me to speak to a group of registered nurses (RNs) at the University of Massachusetts Memorial Health Care Campus in Worcester. Usually, such events are up-beat—occasions for **flowery** praise of America's largest predominantly female profession, which is also the largest profession in the health care system. Not today. The 30 or so middle-aged nurses who **straggle** into a bare auditorium look like they're attending a **wake**.

In a sense, they are. These RNs entered the profession with high expectations and a strong sense of purpose several decades ago, but the field they work in is no longer either patient- or nurse-friendly terrain. The health care system has changed, and nurses like the weary ones at this event feel they are unable to fulfill their historic mission of caring for the sick. "Nurses are simply exhausted," explains Kate Maker, an RN for 16 years who works on an intensive care unit (ICU). "Patients can't survive without our services. But today we can't give them those services" because they are sicker, and there are more patients for each nurse to take care of.

Patient well-being and survival rates are greatly affected by the quality of nursing care. So why are we driving nurses out of the profession?

In the ongoing public debate about the quality of market-driven medicine, most criticism has focused on the deterioration of physician autonomy and of the doctor-patient relationship under **managed care.** But health care cost cutting and competition are having an ever-more damaging impact not just on doctors but on the nation's 2.6 million RNs.

Hospital restructurings and down-sizings have slashed bedside nursing staff—the backbone of the hospital—and have replaced RNs with poorly trained and poorly paid **nursing assistants.** Those RNs who remain at the bedside must now care for greater numbers of sicker patients who are assembly-lined through the hospital in shorter and shorter periods of time. Ironically, in an era when much attention is focused on the problem of **medical errors,** nurses no longer have time to be patients' 24-hours-a-day early-warning and early-intervention system. They no longer have time to get to know patients and respond to their needs. Even as the medical system as a whole becomes increasingly impersonal, nurses can no longer provide the level of comfort and compassion they once did.

The consequences of cuts in nursing care are extremely serious. Patients who could recover, don't. **Preventable complications** escalate. Some patients die. Moreover, as nurses are stretched

flowery—overflowing **straggle**—walk in a tired way **wake**—funeral

too thin in the hospital and as patients are denied expert nursing care at home, the burden of care is shifted to unpaid, ill-prepared family caregivers.

Largely because of current conditions, veteran nurses are leaving the field and potential new entrants are being discouraged from joining the profession. Just as the population is aging and in need of more nursing care, the nation now faces a new nursing shortage.

More Patients, Fewer Nurses

As hospitals compete for managed care contracts and try to gain **clout** with insurers, cost cutting is moving more and more money away from the bedside. Faced with lower fees from both **HMOs** and **Medicare,** hospitals are desperate to save money. Since RNs represent 23 percent of the hospital workforce and are the biggest share of labor costs (and are only 10 percent unionized), downsizing RN staff has become an irresistible cost-reduction strategy.

Over the past decade, hospitals have turned to expensive consultants who assure anxious hospital CEOs that their product is just like any other easily definable, measurable **commodity**. Change the production process, make operations more efficient, replace expensive employees with cheaper ones, and help those who remain to be more productive—you'll save money without sacrificing quality, consultants say.

Hospitals have thus downsized their RN staffs through layoffs or by attrition. They have also replaced RNs, who in 1996 earned on average $37,738 plus benefits, with unlicensed assistive personnel (UAPs), who earn 20 to 40 percent less.

No states regulate the education of nurse assistants. So someone without a high school diploma and a few hours of on-the-job training may change **sterile** dressings, **insert urinary catheters,** or **clean tracheotomy** tubes. Meanwhile these nursing assistants are actually practicing under the supervising RN's license; under state licensure rules, the RN can be held responsible for any mistakes made by aides working under his or her direction—and can lose his or her license as a result of those mistakes.

To make sure workers are productive, hospitals may also cross-train janitors, housekeepers, transport workers, and security guards to do nursing work. (That person changing your tracheotomy tube may be a janitor!) Studies report that hospital nursing staffs, which once consisted of 85–95 percent registered nurses and only 5–15 percent aides, are now only 80, 70—sometimes 50—percent registered nurses and up to 50 percent aides.

Hospitals often dispute nurses' claims that restructuring has resulted in fewer nurses at the bedside. The American Hospital Association (AHA), for example, contends that the number of RNs employed in hospitals actually rose from 858,909 in 1992, to 901,198 in 1997. But the association does not take account of where in the hospitals RNs are working. Hospitals provide the AHA only with aggregate FTEs (full-time equivalent positions), a number that includes all RNs regardless of whether they're involved in providing direct care or have purely administrative functions, such as dealing with insurance companies.

"Hospitals now have a **cadre** of RNs who are taking care of the **charts,** not the patients," says Jean Chaisson, a clinical nurse specialist at the Beth Israel Deaconess Medical Center in Boston. "On a floor with fewer RNs spread thinner, when I'm busy rushing one patient to the **operating room,** these **case managers** or **utilization reviewers** are not there to help make sure another patient isn't falling on the floor."

---

clout—influence **commodity**—something that can be bought or sold **cadre**—group

Besides, even according to the AHA's own statistics, when RN FTEs are calculated on a per-admission basis—reflecting the volume of patients and intensity of the patients' needs—their number declines slightly. This report explains that there are "fewer RNs particularly in markets with high managed care penetration."

Nurses like Chaisson tell us that their workload has increased and that they may be taking care of two or three times the number of patients they took care of in the past—perhaps 10 to 16 patients on **medical surgical floors** or three to four patients in ICUs.

The Institute for Health and Socio-Economic Policy (IHSP) recently analyzed 18.2 million California hospital **discharge records** and other data collected from state agencies and the hospital industry for the California Nurses Association. Between 1994 and 1997, there was an 8.8 percent increase in the average number of patients for which an RN cared, a 7.2 percent decrease in the number of RNs employed, and a 7.7 percent jump in the number of patients per **staffed bed** between 1995 and 1998.

The New York State Nurses Association reported similar findings when it surveyed its state's RNs. Twenty-two percent of the nurses who responded said they were responsible for 10 or more patients. Hospital **surgical nurses** reported an average patient load of 9.4 patients, and **critical care nurses,** 3.14 patients. Forty-six percent of the nurses said they couldn't provide the level of nursing care patients needed.

What Jane Smith faces when she gets to work at night on an **orthopedic** floor in a southern community hospital is typical for today's restructured nurse. (Note: Some of the names in this article have been changed.) With only one aide, she routinely cares for up to 20 **frail**, elderly patients who have just emerged from the operating room after having **total hip** or **knee replacements.** Her patients are completely immobilized and may be in excruciating pain. Smith has to take their vital signs frequently, **draw** their **blood,** and every few hours **inject drugs** (such as **pain relievers,** or heart or ulcer medications) into their veins.

It is now well known that insufficient pain medication **jeopardizes** a patient's ability to heal. It is also well known that pain medication should be administered well before patients are turned or do their **physical therapy.** But Smith says, "If you have a really heavy patient load, you don't have time to do it. They ask for pain medication, and I tell them I'll be there as soon as I can. I recently had five patients in a row who needed **meds,** and I had to put them on a list. You run in there and give them meds, and get a **pain scale,** and ask if there's anything you can do and they'll say, 'You're too busy. I don't want to ask you.'"

Orthopedic **surgeon** William Marshall works with Jane Smith and shares her frustrations. Because nurses are so overloaded, he says, "you order a **unit of blood** at 6:30 in the morning, and you find out that at 5:30 in the evening it still has not been given. You find patients [who were] calling for medicine for pain, and it wasn't given to them until an hour-and-a-half later.

Marshall says that "cuts to the bone" are driving individual nurses to despair. "There are people with whom I've worked for 10 or 15 years," he explains with mounting distress, "and I find them in tears, saying, 'I can't stand it anymore. I'm going to leave.'"

Sicker Patients, Busier Nurses

Another cost-cutting measure—shortened length of hospital stay—is changing the nature of patient needs and making it more difficult for nurses to minister to them.

---

frail—weak

For almost every operation, treatment, or diagnostic procedure requiring hospitalization, length of stay has been shortened. Although getting patients out of the hospital and back home is **touted** as a wonderful thing for patients, it actually makes it harder to care for those who are hospitalized.

In the past, people came into the hospital for surgery the day before their operations and stayed in the hospital until they were well on the road to **recovery.** Today, the 91-year-old woman who is on Jane Smith's unit (after a hip replacement operation) does not come in the day before surgery for **tests,** but arrives at the hospital on the day of the operation. Nor will the woman remain in the hospital until she recovers. She's out in three days. Which means she is much sicker while she's in the hospital, as are all the other patients nurses care for.

When length of stay is so truncated, the hospital becomes like a Midas **muffler** shop. Forty to 50 percent of the total patients admitted to a hospital may be discharged in 24 hours. Barbara Norrish of the Samuel Merritt College Department of Nursing and Thomas Rundall of the University of California–Berkeley's School of Public Health have demonstrated that patients' shortened length of stay increases nurses' cumulative **patient load.** "A typical nurse may come onto her unit at 7:00 in the morning and take care of seven patients with an aide," says Norrish. "But four of those patients are discharged at noon, and four new patients are admitted at 1:00 PM. The nurse manager who sees the patients at 1:00 PM will argue that the nurse only has seven patients. But she doesn't; she has 11."

Plus with all these **admissions** and discharges, activity on the unit—not just at the bedside—also escalates with nurses spending as much time talking to **home care agencies, rehabilitation facilities, nursing homes,** or family members, negotiating the **hand-off** of the patient, as they do for **direct patient care.**

Erica Wilson, who works in an oncology clinic in a prestigious teaching hospital in a major metropolitan area in the Northeast, is a case in point. In her clinic, the same number of RNs now see more patients than ever before. Half of Wilson's patients are on experimental treatments. She must spend more time reviewing treatment plans and double-checking **calculations** of **drug dosages.** Because the side effects of **experimental drugs** aren't well known, those drugs must be **infused** more slowly. Wilson also has to closely monitor patients, respond to any hint of an **adverse reaction,** and review with patients complex schedules for chemotherapy.

Many of her patients now take highly **toxic** drugs—drugs that used to be administered in a hospital or clinic—at home. If they experience side effects, they call the clinic. Wilson must leave patients to respond to these calls. At the same time, patients who have been discharged from the hospital while they are still ill are bringing more serious problems to the clinic. And the increased volume of sicker patients leads to more clinic emergencies like cardiac and respiratory arrests. As a result of the volume and **acuity** of patients, "things are being missed," she says. "If we aren't making major mistakes, it's **by the skin of our teeth.**"

The consequences of cuts in nursing care are extremely serious. Patients who could recover, don't. Complications escalate. Patients die.

Such heavy caseloads don't only detract from patient care; they erode the quality of the nurses' working life. **Harried** RNs say they have no time to go to the bathroom, eat lunch, or have a cup of coffee much less get off the unit to attend essential educational seminars.

---

touted—advertised **muffler**—exhaust pipe for a car **Harried** —under pressure

One stressed-out emergency room nurse explains that she has more than once almost fainted because she can't find a moment in her eight-hour shift to get a bite to eat. Another RN tells me she won't drink tea or coffee on the job because caffeine just makes her go to the bathroom, and she has no time to take a toilet break. More say they suffer from stress-related illnesses, like ulcers, **colitis,** and **hypertension.** Because they are unable to get help turning and moving patients, many report back **injuries**.

According to the Bureau of Labor Statistics, 700,000 health care workers suffered an injury or illness in 1996—twice as many as were reported in 1990. The rate of injuries surpassed that of manufacturing, construction, and mining, which are well-known high-hazard industries. Of the 91 categories of workers the Bureau of Labor Statistics measures, RNs ranked fourth in days lost at work due to **nonfatal** illnesses and injuries. Only "stock handlers and baggers," "freight and stock material handlers" and "laborers/construction workers"—all primarily male—had more illnesses and injuries. In Minnesota, between 1990 and 1994, when restructuring efforts reduced nursing by 9.2 percent, there was a 65 percent increase in RN work-related injuries and illnesses.

Nurses' morale is also plummeting because of an increased use of **"floating"** and **mandatory** overtime, scheduling practices that nurses have long **deplored** as unsafe to patients and demeaning to nurses. When nurses float, they are moved from the unit where they usually work to one with which they may not be familiar. For example, if a cardiac nurse calls in sick or goes on vacation, managers may send an oncology nurse to replace him or her. "Would you ask an ear, nose, and throat doctor or dermatologist to cover cardiology for the day and expect high quality care?" Jean Chaisson asks. "I don't think so."

Today, after an exhausting 8- or 12-hour shift, a nurse may also suddenly learn that he or she has to work an extra 8 or 12 hours. For a largely female workforce with child care and family responsibilities, this is particularly **onerous**.

"You work from 3:00 in the afternoon to 11:00 at night. You have arranged for someone to take care of your kids," says Kate Maker, a nurse at the University of Massachusetts Medical Center in Worcester. "So at 10:00 you're told you have to work mandatory overtime. Well, just like the hospital can't pull nurses out of the sky to suddenly work 11 to 7, we can't pull babysitters out of the sky at 11:00 at night to take care of our kids. We're put in the terrible position of having to choose between abandoning our patients and abandoning our children." If RNs protest that these assignments are unsafe for their patients, they are often warned that refusing the assignments will constitute **"patient abandonment"**—a charge that can lead to a disciplinary action by the state Board of Registration in Nursing.

Perhaps more than anything else, nursing morale has bottomed out because RNs say they no longer have time to really "care" for their patients. "Before, I was able to sit in a room and teach patients about their care and listen to them," an ICU nurse in the Midwest told me. "But today, you can't have any kind of interaction with patients. You don't have time to talk with them, or hold their hand, or be with them. Today, we only have time to take care of their tubes." This nurse eventually left the hospital.

Losing Nurses, Losing Lives

Not surprisingly, patients and their family members are feeling the side effects of the disorganization of nursing care. Madge Kaplan is the Boston-based Health Desk editor for National Public Radio's Marketplace show. Last winter, her 81-year-old father had a **stroke** and was hospitalized at a major northeastern teaching hospital. He then spent a total of three months in its **inpatient** and rehabilitation units. The medical aspects of his care, Kaplan explains, were excellent.

But Kaplan adds, "If my father or the three other patients in his room needed to go to the bathroom, if they needed to reposition themselves to eat a meal, if they needed help in adjusting their

---

deplored—condemned **onerous**—burdensome

position in a wheelchair, if they needed help unwrapping utensils to eat a meal, that help was not forthcoming."

It was "tragic," Kaplan says, to watch "these frightened, frail elderly patients push themselves to the limit of their energy to get someone to pay attention to them. Pleading with someone to get a glass of water or to wipe someone up when they had spilled something on their bed."

Kaplan, like Jane Smith's patients, understood that the nursing staff were overwhelmed. "Nurses seemed to have their hands full—so much so that I always came away feeling that staff seemed tense, stretched, and in no mood to engage with patients and the people visiting them." Although boosters of market-driven health care insist that "consumers" like Kaplan and her father will vigorously advocate for themselves when they don't get the service they expect, neither complained to hospital administration. Why? Because when people are sick, vulnerable, and totally dependent, they are loath to alienate those who hold their lives in their hands.

Patients do, however, register their concerns when they are not immediately dependent on their hospital for care. In 1996, the AHA sent its members a confidential report entitled "Reality Check: Public Perceptions of Health Care and Hospitals." The report summarized data gathered in focus groups with 300 patients in 12 states plus an opinion survey of another 1,000 patients. "The key indicator that people referred to as a measure of quality of their hospital care" the report stated, "was the nurse." The report went on to say that those surveyed

> hold a strong belief that skilled nurses are being systematically replaced by poorly trained and poorly paid aides. Their perspective on the "thinness" of hospital nurse staffing was reflected in a universally mentioned experience: "If I hadn't stayed in the hospital room with my mother, child, or spouse, they would never have gotten the correct medication or care on time." People believe the profit motive is behind the reduction in nursing care. They are angry at the reversal in health care priorities this represents.

In the face of patient and nurse complaints, the hospital and insurance industries often argue that nurses have not proven their worth and that their critical role in patient care has not been scientifically documented.

Nothing could be further from the truth. While nursing's contributions—like those of other predominantly female occupations—have hardly received the kind of research attention devoted to the highly male medical profession, there is, in fact, a considerable body of scientific literature that explains what nurses do and why it is critical to patient health.

Jeffrey H. Silber and his colleagues at the University of Pennsylvania School of Medicine are studying an important variable in determining patient mortality—what they call **"failure to rescue."** These researchers report that among hospitals with comparably adjusted case mixes, some are better at "rescuing" patients than others. Working with researchers Linda Aiken and Julie Sochalski of the University of Pennsylvania School of Nursing, they have identified the critical factors in patient rescue. Hospitals need to have enough educated staff who recognize a problem when they see it. Those staff must be with patients enough of the time and must have enough status and authority in the institution to mobilize resources and deal with crises. Nurses, the researchers explain, are the educated eyes-on/hands-on, 24-hour-**surveillance**-and-intervention system in hospitals.

When, as other recent studies confirm, hospitals employ enough educated nurses and give them ample time with patients, patients have fewer urinary tract **infections, falls, pneumonias,** and **bedsores.** And they are less likely to die. When Aiken and her colleagues analyzed the care of AIDS

---

surveillance—observation

patients, they documented that "an additional 0.5 nurse per patient per day—or an additional nurse for every six patients on each eight-hour shift—would be expected to reduce the likelihood of [patients] dying by roughly one-third."

In October, Michael Rie, an **anesthesiologist** and **intensive care physician** at the University of Kentucky, presented a quality-assurance analysis of ICU **re-admissions** in one university hospital. (The data were collected in response to findings that the average length of ICU stay for patients with respiratory problems was longer than that suggested by a nationally accepted benchmark.) The study found that patients at low risk of death and/or re-admission to ICU—who had been discharged to regular hospital floors—were being re-admitted at a seemingly elevated rate. Patients with a predicted low risk of death, 10 percent, had an actual mortality rate of 24 percent.

When investigators explored why patients were readmitted to the ICU, they discovered that 80 percent of these patients had potentially preventable ICU re-admissions. The problem was they weren't receiving enough basic respiratory care on non-ICU floors. A plausible inference is that there weren't enough staff in this hospital to **suction** patients' lungs and help them cough.

Not only is this endangering patients' health and sometimes their lives; it's not even cost-effective. In this particular hospital, for example, the non-labor costs for the ICU re-admission of only 79 patients was $1.6 million—or 35 percent of the cost of their entire hospitalization. If labor costs were added to this figure, it would be two to three times as high. (This points to the need not just for better staffing but also for **intermediate care units** that provide a level of services less intensive than in ICUs but more intensive than on **general care floors.**) The fact that cutting nursing services doesn't save money is confirmed in other studies about hospital restructuring.

Laying off RNs and replacing them with aides works only for so long. Eventually hospitals have to hire additional RNs. But today, when they try to fill vacancies, many hospitals are finding it more and more difficult to attract new recruits. In a report on the new nursing shortage, even the AHA concludes that "RN Dissatisfaction May Be Driving the Current Shortage in Hospitals."

This increasingly well-publicized dissatisfaction with working conditions and concern about the quality of patient care is driving young women and men away from studying nursing in the first place. In an era of low unemployment, especially when women have more career options than ever before, why would anyone want to spend the time and money involved in getting a nursing education for the privilege of being part of a cheap, disposable labor force? And why would more men decide to enter a "women's profession" that even women are finding unattractive? It is hardly surprising that the number of young people interested in entering four-year nursing programs has been steadily declining over the past four years and fell by 5.5 percent in 1998.

What Can Be Done

Nurses have tried to focus public attention on the erosion of their working conditions. In [2000] both Massachusetts and California passed whistle-blower bills. And after intense pressure from the California Nurses Association, [then] California Governor Gray Davis signed the first safe-staffing law anywhere in the country (and he did it despite the opposition of the state's hospital industry). In response to this measure, hospitals must comply with the new nurse-to-patient ratios by 2007 and limit the floating of nurses between units.

But while legislation like California's can help alleviate the nation's persistent nursing crisis, it is only a short-term solution. Many other, more fundamental changes need to be made in both the financing and delivery of health care. As long as we have a job-based, employer-dominated private health insurance system in which billions of dollars are siphoned off every year for unnecessary advertising, marketing, and administrative costs (not to mention insurance and drug company profiteering), those who provide hands-on care will always be starved for resources.

But though national health insurance is a necessary first step toward improvement, it is not in itself a sufficient condition for quality nursing care. Even if America eventually provides tax-supported coverage as Canadians have had since the 1970s, nursing care may still be a cost-cutting target (as it has been in Canada lately) if the value that nurses add to the health care system is not recognized.

In other words, despite recent curbs on physician autonomy and specialist referrals, most people—even under the degraded conditions of managed care—regard *medically necessary care* as an entitlement. There is, however, no parallel conception of *necessary nursing care*. If such a concept did exist, the training and deployment of nurses and the organization of nursing care within hospitals would be seen as no less important to patient outcomes than medicine's role in diagnosis and treatment. The dangers of both radically reduced hospital stays and insufficient nursing care in other settings would be more widely understood. And there would be better pay for and treatment of nurses as well as greater social recognition and respect.

Our contract with RNs would be, in effect, that we must care about them if we want *them* to care for us.

Activity: Vocabulary Development

Reading 2.2 contains many specialized medical/nursing terms. Add the words you do not know to your dictionary, following the guidelines on page 33. Use a medical English dictionary to look up the specialized terms you do not know. Use 10–15 new words in answering the discussion questions.

Comprehension and Discussion Questions

These questions ask you to locate important information in Reading 2.2, as well as analyze carefully and think critically about information in the reading. In small groups, discuss your answers.

1. How has the patient workload changed in recent years? Provide data from the Institute for Health and Socio-Economic Policy (IHSP) to support your answer. According to the New York State Nurses Association, what is the average patient load? For a surgical nurse? For a critical care nurse? How has the increase in patient workload affected the care of patients?
2. What is a "Midas muffler shop"? What does the author mean by "the hospital becomes like a Midas muffler shop" (page 49)? How has the "shortened length of hospital stay" (page 49) affected the care of patients and the working conditions of nurses?

3. What is "failure to rescue" (page 51)? What are the critical factors in patient rescue, according to research studies by Silber and his colleagues at the University of Pennsylvania School of Medicine and the School of Nursing? Why are these findings especially significant within the context of a nursing crisis?
4. Besides patient rescue, in what other ways has quality of nursing care been linked to patient recovery?
5. According to this article, what are the reasons for the new nursing shortage?
6. What is a "whistle-blower" (page 52) bill? What are the provisions of the "first safe-staffing law" (page 52) in nursing that passed in California a few years ago?
7. According to Gordon, are such legislative measures sufficient to solve "the nation's persistent nursing crisis" (page 52)? In her view, what measures are necessary to ensure long-term quality nursing care?
8. Now that you have read the article and answered the above questions, what do you think was Gordon's purpose in writing this article? Provide support for your answer. Was the author effective in accomplishing her intended purpose? Why or why not?
9. How does this article differ in content and style from Gordon's first article that you read, "Caring Means Curing" (Unit 1, Reading 1.2)?
10. How does this article by Gordon differ in content and style from "The Evolution of a Crisis: Nursing in America" by Kimball and O'Neil (Reading 2.1 in this unit)?

Reading and Interpreting Figures

Information in readings is sometimes displayed in visual form, that is, as a table or figure. **Tables** display numerical information, usually in columns. **Figures** display information in some other format, such as a **graph** or **diagram,** and are usually some combination of numerical and nonnumerical information. A **graph** shows the relationship between two variables and is organized along **horizontal and vertical axes.** A **diagram** is a drawing that shows how something works or what something looks like.

Tables and figures are often used to support information in a text, so if you are unable to read and correctly interpret the table or figure, you may not understand the information in the reading.

The focus in Reading 2.3, " Nursing in the Crossfire," is on understanding figures. Preview the figures, and answer the questions.

Look at **Figure 1:**

Figure 1 Levels of Staffing by Nurses in Registered Community Hospitals in the United States, 1983 to 2000

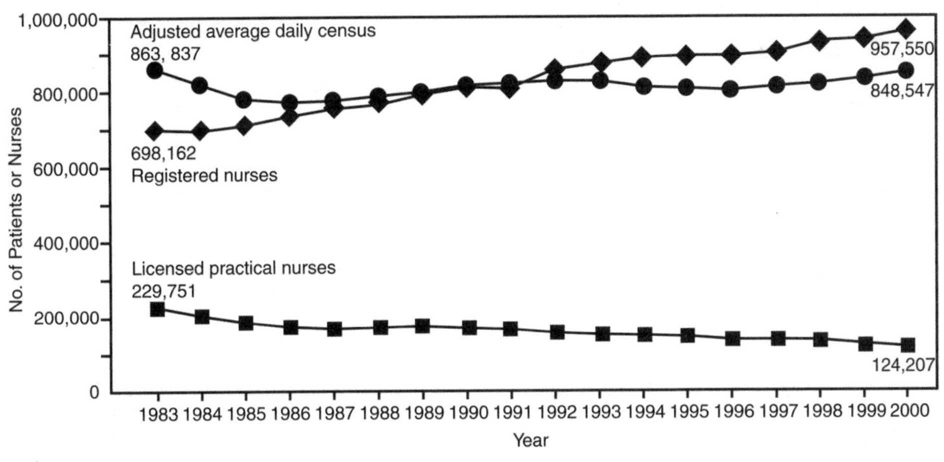

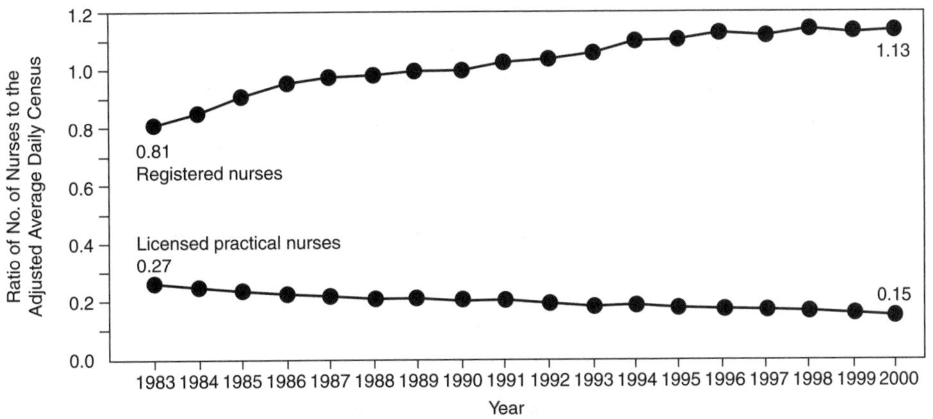

Source: Data are from the American Hospital Association, Health Forum, AHA Annual Survey of Hospitals, 1983–2000.

This figure consists of two separate, but related figures. First of all, preview the figure: What do the units along the *horizontal axis* in *both* figures represent? ____________ What size are the increments? ____________ What do the units along the *vertical axis* in the *top* figure represent? ____________ What size are the increments? ____________ What do the units along the *vertical axis* in the *bottom* figure represent? ____________ What size are the increments? ____________

Answer the questions.

1. In what year did the number of hospitalized patients and the number of registered nurses overlap the most? ____________________

2. Has there been an overall increase or decrease in the number of hospitalized patients from 1983 to 2000? ____________________

   By how many? ____________________

   ____

3. Has there been an overall increase or decrease in the number of registered nurses from 1983 to 2000? ____________________

   By how many? ____________________

4. Has there been an overall increase or decrease in the ratio of nurses to patients? ____________________

   By how much? ____________________

   Given your answer for Question 3, Reading 2.2, did you expect this?

   ____

   Why or why not? ____________________

   ____

5. In your own words, tell what this figure is showing you. ____________________

   ____

Read the text that refers to Figure 1. Did it help to have studied the figure before reading the text? Why or why not?

Between 1983 and 2000, the staffing levels of registered nurses in hospitals increased by 37 percent (Figure 1). The staffing levels of licensed practical nurses decreased by 46 percent. The average daily census of hospitalized patients fluctuated but decreased overall. Through 1993, the ratio of registered nurses to patients increased, but it may merely have kept pace with increases in the severity of patients' conditions.[11] Although the ratio of registered nurses to hospitalized patients remained relatively constant between 1994 and 2000, there are no recent data on staffing that adjust for the severity of patients' illnesses as well as their shorter lengths of stay.

In Figure 1, absolute numbers are shown in the top panel, and ratios in the lower panel. The number of registered nurses and the ratio of registered nurses to patients have increased. The number of hospitalized patients, the number of licensed practical nurses and the ratio of licensed practical nurses to patients have decreased. The number of registered nurses and the number of licensed practical nurses shown are full-time equivalents. The adjusted average daily census was calculated by dividing the number of inpatient-days by the number of days in the reporting period. Registered community hospitals (short-term general and specialty hospitals that are registered with the American Hospital Association) are included; federal hospitals are not included. Data are from the American Hospital Association, Health Forum, AHA Annual Survey of Hospitals, 1983–2000.

[11] Aiken, L. H., Sochalski, J., & Anderson, G. F. (1996). Downsizing the hospital nursing workforce. *Health Affairs, 15* (11), 88–92.

Look at **Figure 2:**

Figure 2 Actual and Inflation-Adjusted Average Annual Salaries of Full-Time Registered Nurses in the United States, 1980 to 2000

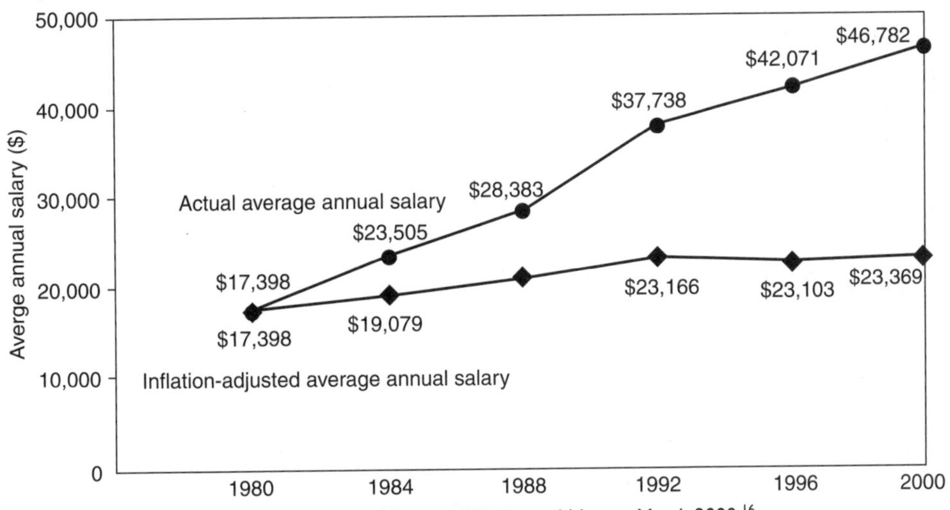

Source: Adapted from the National Sample of Survey of Registered Nurses, March 2000.[16]

What do the units along the *horizontal axis* in the figure represent? ____________ What size are the increments? ____________ What do the units along the *vertical axis* represent? ____________ What size are the increments? ____________ What is the difference between an "actual average annual salary" and an "inflation-adjusted average annual salary"? ______

____

Answer the questions.

1. In **Figure 2,** what is the difference in dollar amount between the "actual average annual salary" from 1980 to 2000? ____________
2. What is the difference in dollar amount between the "inflation-adjusted average annual salary" from 1980 to 2000? ____________
3. In your opinion, do full-time registered nurses make a decent income? ____________
4. In your own words, tell what this figure is showing you. ____________

____

[16]Spratley et al.

Read the text that refers to Figure 2. Did it help to have studied the figure before reading the text? Why or why not?

In recent years, wages for registered nurses have been relatively flat as compared with the rate of inflation (Figure 2). In 2000, the average annual salary of a registered nurse employed full-time was $46,782.[16] Between 1980 and 1992, real annual salaries for registered nurses increased by nearly $6,000. Between 1992 and 2000, however, they increased by only about $200.

Look at **Figure 3:**

Figure 3 Enrollment in Educational Programs to Train Registered Nurses in the United States

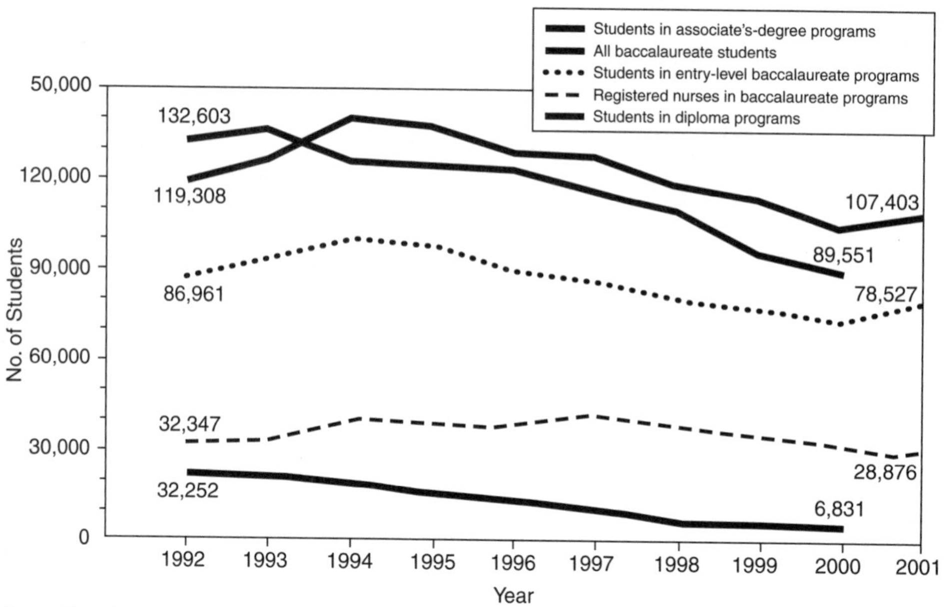

Source: Data for baccalaureate programs are from the American Association of Colleges of Nursing. Data for associate's-degree and diploma programs are from the National League for Nursing.

[16]Spratley, E., Johnson, A., Sochalski, J., Fritz, M., & Spencer, W. (2002, February). *The registered nurse population: Findings from the National Sample Survey of Registered Nurses: March 2000.* Washington, DC: Health Resources and Service Administration.

What do the units along the *horizontal axis* in the figure represent? ____________ What size are the increments? ____________ What do the units along the *vertical axis* represent? ____________ What size are the increments? ____________

Answer the questions.

1. Look at the box in the upper right-hand corner of the figure. How many kinds of nursing programs are there in the United States? ____________
   What are they? ____________
2. In the figure itself, the top line in the upper left-hand corner represents associate's degree students. Has there been an overall increase or decrease in the number of students in associate's degree programs from 1992 to 2001? ____________
   By how many? ____________
3. The second line in the upper left-hand corner of the figure represents all baccalaureate-degree students. Has there been an overall increase or decrease in the number of students in baccalaureate programs from 1992 to 2001? ____________
   By how many? ____________
4. The last line in the lower left-hand corner of the figure represents students in diploma programs. Has there been an overall increase or decrease in the number of students in diploma programs from 1992 to 2001?
   ____
   By how many? ____________
5. Which program(s) experienced an increase in student enrollment from 2000 to 2001? ____________
   Why do you think there was an increase in this type of program? ____________
   ____
6. In your own words, tell what this figure is showing you. ____________
   ____

Read these texts that refer to Figure 3. Did it help to have studied the figure before reading the text? Why or why not?

In the 1990s, the growth of managed care slowed employment growth for registered nurses in hospitals, particularly in states such as California.[22,23] There was a surplus of registered nurses; some nurses lost their jobs, and some new nurses were unable to find jobs. Although hospitals were still hiring more registered nurses (Figure 1), it seemed that they might need fewer in the long term. Enrollment in nursing schools declined (Figure 3).

Enrollment in associate's-degree programs for nurses decreased through 2000, according to preliminary data (Figure 3). One encouraging sign, however, is that enrollment in baccalaureate programs, which appeal to younger students,[77] has increased[78] (Figure 3). The increase — in 2001 — ended a six-year period of declining enrollment.

Look at **Figure 4:**

Figure 4 Employed Registered Nurses per 100,000 Population

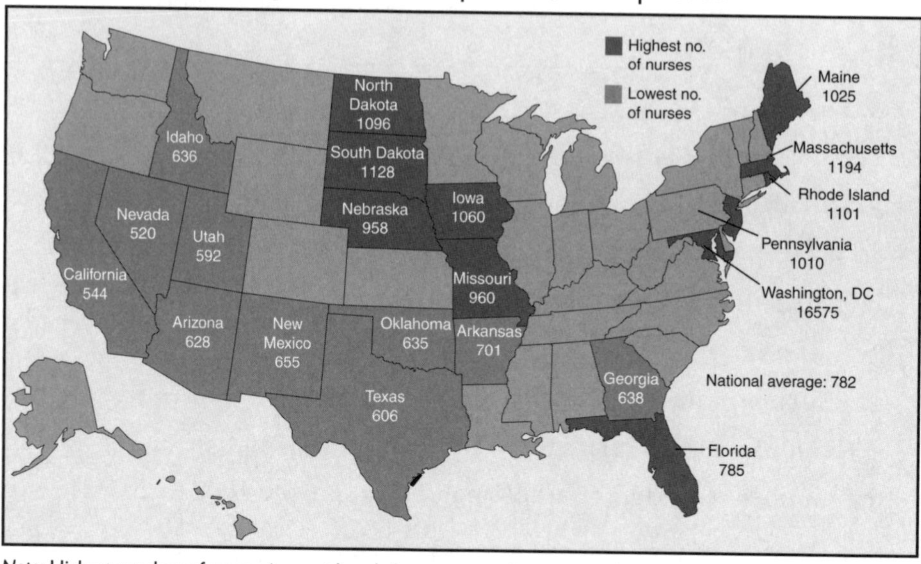

Note: Highest number of nurses is considered above average. Lowest number of nurses is considered below average. Although Florida has an average number of nurses (785) that is slightly above the national average of 782, it is included in the discussion in the article as a state that has a below-average number of nurses.
Source: Data are from the National Sample Survey of Registered Nurses, March 2000.

[22]Buerhaus, P. I., & Staiger, D. O. (1996). Managed care and the nurse workforce. *Journal of the American Medical Association, 276*, 1487–1493.
[23]Buerhaus, P. I., & Staiger, D. O. (1999). Trouble in the nurse labor market? Recent trends and future outlook. *Health Affairs, 18*(1), 214–222.
[77]Auerbach, D. I., Buerhaus, P. I., & Staiger, D. O. (2000). Associate degree graduates and the rapidly aging RN workforce. *Nursing Economics, 18*, 178–184.
[78]*Enrollments rise at U.S. nursing colleges and universities ending a six-year period of decline* (2001, December 20). Press release of the American Association of Colleges of Nursing, Washington, DC.

In this figure, the United States has been divided into two categories. What are those two categories? ____________________ and ____________________.

Answer the questions.

1. What is the national *average* of employed registered nurses per 100,000 population? ____________________
2. What is the state with the *lowest* number of nurses per 100,000 population? ____________________
3. Which of the 50 states has the *highest* number of nurses per 100,000 population? ____________________
4. Which region of the country seems to have the lowest concentration of nurses, based on the numbers provided in this figure? (Northeast, Southeast, Upper Midwest, Lower Midwest, Southwest, Northwest)

   ____

   Which two regions seem to have the highest concentration of nurses?

   ____________________ and ____________________
5. In your own words, tell what this figure is showing you. ____________________

   ____

Read these texts that refer to Figure 4. Did it help to have studied the figure before reading the text? Why or why not?

The number of employed registered nurses per capita varies widely from state to state (Figure 4). In 2000, the national average was 782 employed nurses per 100,000 population. California had only 544, whereas Massachusetts had 1194 and Pennsylvania had 1010.[25] These variations have been cited as evidence of regional shortages of nurses, particularly in states with a low supply of nurses, such as California,[26] Nevada,[27] and Texas.[28] The demand for hospital-based nurses, however, reflects many factors, including the number of hospital beds, the average length of stay, the specific medical services offered, population growth, and the number of elderly residents. Although Florida has 785 nurses per 100,000 population — about the national average — the supply has been considered inadequate because the state has the highest percentage of elderly persons in the nation.[29] Because a low supply of nurses may reflect a low demand — not an unmet demand — for hospital-based nurses, the importance of the variations in and of themselves is uncertain.

In 2001, the mean vacancy rate for registered-nurse positions at a given hospital was 13 percent. Fifteen percent of hospitals reported vacancy rates of 20 percent or more.[31] Mean vacancy rates were 11 percent in the Northeast and Midwest, 13 percent in the South, and 15 percent in the West. There were about 126,000 vacant positions nationwide.[32]

Look at **Figure 5:**

Figure 5 Age Distribution of Registered Nurses in the United States, 1980 through 2000

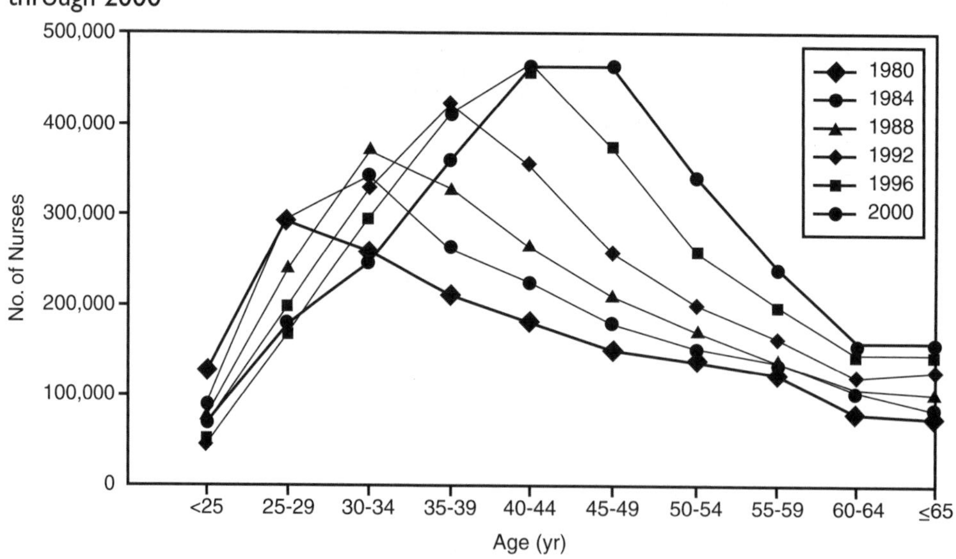

Source: Adapted from the National Sample Survey of Registered Nurses, March 2000.

[25]Spratley et al.

[26]Coffman, J., & Spetz, J. (1999). Maintaining an adequate supply of RNs in California. *Journal of Nursing Scholarship, 31*, 389–393.

[27]Richmond, E. (2002, January, 14). New hospitals face staffing woes: Nursing shortage is 'reaching crisis levels in Nevada.' *Las Vegas Sun*, 1.

[28]Miller, D. R. (2000, Winter). *Health and nurses in Texas: The supply of registered nurses: First look at available data, 1*(1). San Antonio: University of Texas Health Science Center.

[29]*Florida's nursing shortage: It is here and it is getting worse* (2001, November). Orlando: Florida Hospital Association.

[31]*The healthcare workforce shortage and its implications for America's hospitals* (2001, Fall). Long Beach, CA.: First Consulting Group.

[32]*The hospital workforce shortage: Immediate and future* (2001, June). *TrendWatch,* 3(2). Washington, DC: American Hospital Association, 1-8.

What do the units along the *horizontal axis* in the figure represent? ____________ What size are the increments? ____________ What do the units along the *vertical axis* represent? ____________ What size are the increments? ____________

Answer the questions.

1. Look at the box in the upper right-hand corner of the figure. What do the symbols on the different graph lines represent? ________________
   How many different symbols are represented? ____________________
2. Look at the line representing 1980. Which age category has the greatest number of nurses? ____
   Approximately how many nurses are in that category? ____________
3. Look at the line representing 1988. Which age category has the greatest number of nurses? ____
   Approximately how many nurses are in that category? ____________
4. Look at the line representing 1992. Which age category has the greatest number of nurses? ____
   Approximately how many nurses are in that category? ____________
5. Look at the line representing 2000. Which *two* age categories have the greatest number of nurses? ____________ and ____________________
   Approximately how many nurses are in each category? ____________
6. In your own words, tell what is this figure showing you. ____________
   ____

Read the text that refers to Figure 5. Did it help to have previewed the figure before reading the text? Why or why not?

Both the registered-nurse workforce and the general population are rapidly aging. As members of the "baby boom" generation begin to retire, the demand for nurses is expected to increase rapidly.[46] Between 2000 and 2010, the occupation of registered nurse will be one of the five occupations with the greatest growth in the number of jobs, according to the Bureau of Labor Statistics. It is projected that during this period, there will be 1,000,400 job openings for registered nurses, including 561,000 new positions.[47]

Younger nurses are more likely than older nurses to work in hospitals. In 2000, only 9 percent of registered nurses were less than 30 years of age, as compared with 25 percent in 1980 (Figure 5). About a third of registered nurses were 50 years of age or older.[48] A related issue is that nursing, particularly in a hospital, can be physically demanding and lead to occupational injuries, particularly for older nurses.[49] By 2020, a shortage of more than 400,000 registered nurses is possible.[50] One analysis concluded: "The evidence suggests a not-too-distant collision between the aging and shrinking RN workforce and the increasing demand driven (among other things) by the expanding population of Medicare beneficiaries."[51]

---

[46]Buerhaus, P. I., Staiger, D. O., & Auerbach, D. I. (2000). Implications of an aging registered nurse workforce. *JAMA, 283*, 2948–2954.

[47]Hecker, D. E. (2001, November). Occupational employment projections to 2010. *Monthly Labor Review*, 57–84.

[48]Spratley et al.

[49]Wunderlich et al.

[50]Buerhaus et al.

[51]Buerhaus, P. I., Staiger, D. O., & Auerbach, D. I. (2000). Policy responses to an aging registered nurse workforce. *Nursing Economics, 18*, 278–284, 303.

Reading 2.3

Nursing in the Crossfire

Robert Steinbrook, MD

> What is exceptional in nursing is the nature of the work: the continuous and intimate association with pain and not infrequent contact with death.... Not every man or woman would feel themselves able to undertake the duties of a nurse.
>
> Brian Abel-Smith, *A History of the Nursing Profession*[1]

Nursing is an embattled profession. Many nurses who work in hospitals feel that they are overworked and often unable to provide good patient care. The young people who traditionally have embarked on careers in nursing are increasingly choosing other fields, such as medicine or business, in which the pay and working conditions are better. Nurses who begin their careers in hospitals frequently leave for other positions. As the population ages, the demand for nurses is expected to grow rapidly. But because relatively few young people are entering nursing, severe shortages are anticipated by the end of the decade—unless this trend is reversed.

A 1996 Institute of Medicine report concluded that, although higher levels of staffing by nurses in nursing homes were linked to higher-quality care, the overall data for hospitals were not good enough to "isolate a number-of-RNs effect."[2] In this issue of the *Journal,* Needleman and colleagues[3] report that, in the United States, a higher proportion of hours of nursing care provided by registered nurses (registered-nurse–hours) and a greater number of registered-nurse–hours per day are associated with better outcomes for hospitalized patients. Among medical patients, these outcomes were a shorter length of stay and lower rates of urinary tract infection and upper gastrointestinal bleeding. A higher proportion of registered-nurse–hours was also associated with lower rates of pneumonia, of shock or cardiac arrest, and of death from five causes considered together—pneumonia, shock or cardiac arrest, upper gastrointestinal bleeding, sepsis, or deep venous thrombosis. The findings for surgical patients were similar, although fewer significant associations were found. The study found no evidence of an association between a greater number of hours of care per day provided by licensed practical nurses or hours of care per day provided by nurses' aides and better outcomes.

The study by Needleman et al. focuses attention both on the effect of nursing care on health outcomes and on efforts to increase the level of staffing by registered nurses in hospitals[4,5,6]; such efforts include instituting minimal staffing ratios and prohibiting mandatory overtime, except in emergencies. In this report, I discuss some of the key issues for the nursing profession.

---

[1]Abel-Smith, B. (1960). *A history of the nursing profession.* New York: Springer.

[2]Wunderlich, G. S., Sloan, F. A., & David, C. K. (Eds.). *Nursing staff in hospitals and nursing homes: Is it adequate?* Washington, DC: National Academy Press.

[3]Needleman, J., Buerhaus, P., Mattke, S., Stewart, M., & Zelevinsky, K. (2002). Nurse-staffing levels and the quality of care in hospitals. *New England Journal of Medicine*, 1715–1722.

[4]Freudenheim, M., & Villarosa, L. (2001, April 8). Nursing shortage is raising worries on patients' care. *New York Times*, A1.

[5]Barnard, A. (2002, February 7). As their numbers shrink, nurses gain clout. *Boston Globe*, A1, A28.

[6]Coffman, J., Spetz, J., Seago, J. A., Rosenoff, E., & O'Neil, E. (2001, January). *Nursing in California: A workforce crisis.* San Francisco: California Workforce Initiative.

Background

The problems facing registered nurses are long-standing.[7,8] Registered nurses represent the largest single health care profession in the United States. People usually become registered nurses by completing an associate's-degree program at a community college, a diploma program administered at a hospital, or a baccalaureate degree program at a college or university and then obtaining a state license. During the past 25 years, the number of diploma programs has sharply declined. A 2000 survey of registered nurses who had recently completed their initial nursing education showed that more than half had graduated from an associate's-degree program and about two fifths from a baccalaureate program.[9] Licensed practical nurses account for about one quarter of the nurse work force. They typically have a high-school diploma and are trained in a one-year program at a technical or vocational school or a community or junior college.

Every four years, the National Sample Survey of Registered Nurses provides a statistical snapshot of the profession.[9] In 2000, there were an estimated 2,694,540 persons with a license to practice as registered nurses in the United States. An estimated 82 percent were employed in nursing, and of these, 28 percent were working on a part-time basis. Of the registered nurses employed in nursing, 1,300,323 (59 percent) worked in hospitals. The unemployment rate for registered nurses was about 1 percent.[10] An estimated 95 percent of the nurses were women, 72 percent were married, and 87 percent were white. Their average age was 45 years. Thirty-four percent reported their highest level of education as an associate's degree, 22 percent as graduation from a nursing diploma program, 33 percent as a bachelor's degree, and 10 percent as a master's or doctoral degree. Seven percent were practicing or prepared to practice in an advanced practice role, such as clinical nurse specialist, nurse anesthetist, nurse midwife, or nurse practitioner.

Between 1983 and 2000, the staffing levels of registered nurses in hospitals increased by 37 percent (Figure 1). The staffing levels of licensed practical nurses decreased by 46 percent. The average daily census of hospitalized patients fluctuated but decreased overall. Through 1993, the ratio of registered nurses to patients increased, but it may merely have kept pace with increases in the severity of patients' conditions.[11] Although the ratio of registered nurses to hospitalized patients remained relatively constant between 1994 and 2000, there are no recent data on staffing that adjust for the severity of patients' illnesses as well as their shorter lengths of stay.

Dissatisfaction among Nurses

Nursing "is a very stressful job with a very flat career path," according to Frank Sloan of Duke University, who was the cochair of the committee of the Institute of Medicine that reported on nursing in 1996.[12] "Women are finding many other choices." Registered nurses are discontented for many reasons, including inadequate levels of staffing for both nurses and support staff and excessive workloads. Because hospitalizations are shorter, nurses spend a higher percentage of their time admitting and discharging patients and teaching them what they need to do after they go home. The discontent is part of a broader malaise that also affects physicians and others who work in hospitals.

---

[7]Aiken, L. H., & Mullinix, C. F. (1987). The nurse shortage: Myth or reality? *New England Journal of Medicine, 317*, 641–646.

[8]Iglehart, J. K. (1987). Problems facing the nursing profession. *New England Journal of Medicine, 317*, 646–651.

[9]Spratley, E., Johnson, A., Sochalski, J., Fritz, M., & Spencer, W. (2002, February). *The registered nurse population: Findings from the National Sample Survey of Registered Nurses: March 2000.* Washington, DC: Health Resources and Service Administration.

[10]*Nursing workforce: Emerging nurse shortages due to multiple factors* (2001, July). Washington, DC: General Accounting Office (GAO-01-944).

[11]Aiken, L. H., Sochalski, J., & Anderson, G. F. (1996). Downsizing the hospital nursing workforce. *Health Affairs, 15* (11), 88–92.

[12]Wunderlich, Sloan, & David.

According to the April 2002 report of the American Hospital Association's Commission on Workforce for Hospitals and Health Systems, "Most health care workers entered their professions to 'make a difference' through personal interaction with people in need. Today, many in direct patient care feel tired and burned-out from a stressful, often understaffed environment, with little or no time to experience the one-on-one caring that should be the heart of hospital employment."[13]

Figure 1 Levels of Staffing by Nurses in Registered Community Hospitals in the United States, 1983 to 2000

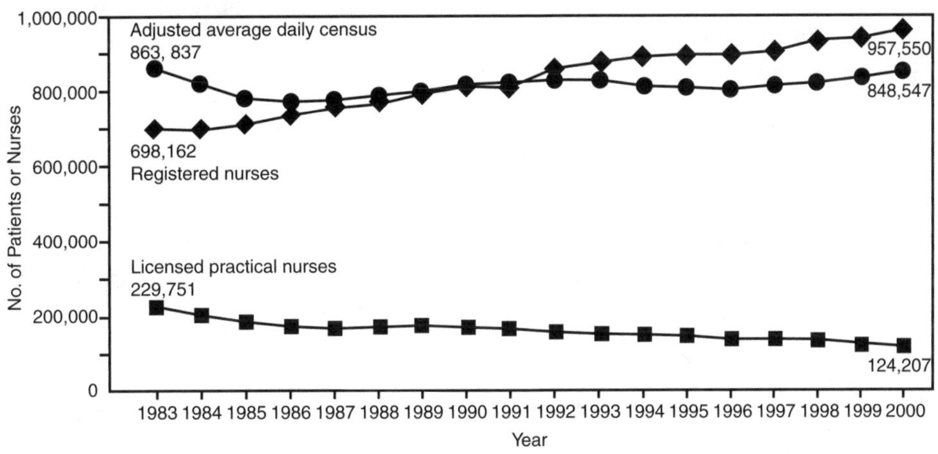

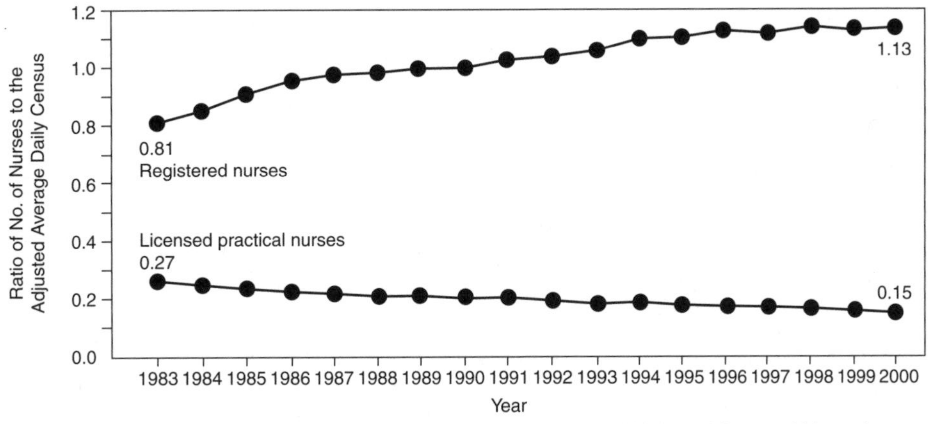

Source: Data are from the American Hospital Association, Health Forum, AHA Annual Survey of Hospitals, 1983–2000.

According to Linda H. Aiken of the University of Pennsylvania School of Nursing, "There is the sense that nursing is becoming an impossible job, and that nurses have no control over things that are required to provide good patient care. Yet nurses are accountable for the health and welfare of

[13]AHA Commission on Workforce for Hospitals and Health Systems (2002, April). *In our hands: How hospital leaders can build a thriving workforce.* Chicago: American Hospital Association.

their patients." The perception is that physicians and hospital administrators often treat registered nurses as workers, not as clinicians and peers, and when possible seek to replace them with less skilled and cheaper personnel, such as licensed practical nurses and aides.

Nurses who begin their careers in hospitals frequently leave for other positions. A large survey of nurses in Pennsylvania, conducted in 1998 and 1999, found that 41 percent were dissatisfied with their present job and that 23 percent of those surveyed were planning to leave this job within the next year.[14] Only about a third agreed with the statements that "there are enough registered nurses to provide high-quality care," "there are enough staff to get the work done," and "the administration listens and responds to nurses' concerns." In a national survey of working nurses conducted in 2001 and 2002, 29 percent of the respondents said they were dissatisfied with their current position; 23 percent were dissatisfied with being a nurse.[15]

Financial Issues

In recent years, wages for registered nurses have been relatively flat as compared with the rate of inflation (Figure 2). In 2000, the average annual salary of a registered nurse employed full-time was $46,782.[16] Between 1980 and 1992, real annual salaries for registered nurses increased by nearly $6,000. Between 1992 and 2000, however, they increased by only about $200.

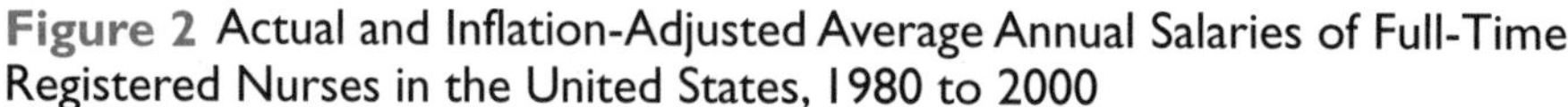

Figure 2 Actual and Inflation-Adjusted Average Annual Salaries of Full-Time Registered Nurses in the United States, 1980 to 2000

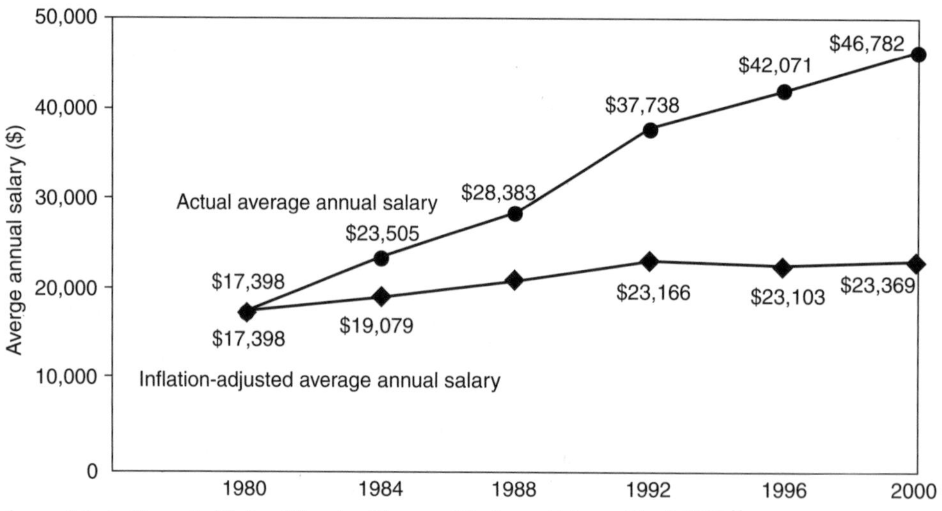

Source: Adapted from the National Sample of Survey of Registered Nurses, March 2000.[16]

[14]Aiken, L. H., Clarke, S. P., & Sloane, D. M., et al. (2001). Nurses' reports on hospital care in five countries. *Health Affairs, 20*(3), 43–53.

[15]NurseWeek/American Organization of Nurse Executives (2002, April). National Survey of Registered Nurses. Sunnyvale, CA: *NurseWeek Publishing*. (Retrieved May 10, 2002, from http://www.nurseweek.com/survey.)

[16]Spratley et al.

Organizing Nurses

Working conditions have been a key issue in recent nursing strikes,[17] such as a bitter two-month strike at the Oregon Health and Science University that ended in February.[18] The ferment within the profession has led to increased interest in collective bargaining. For example, the California Nurses Association has an alliance with the United Steelworkers union. In 2000, 17 percent of registered nurses who were employed in nursing were members of a union, and 19 percent were covered by a collective bargaining agreement.[19] Although these percentages are similar to those for 1990 and 1995, the number of union members has increased—from about 275,000 in 1990 to about 350,000 in 2000—because of the growth in the number of nurses.

There is also a schism between two groups that represent registered nurses. The American Nurses Association, the largest group, has been criticized for being too moderate. The California Nurses Association, a particularly aggressive and politically active group, left the American Nurses Association in 1995. The Massachusetts Nurses Association left in 2001. State nurses associations in California, Massachusetts, Maine, Missouri, and Pennsylvania are forming a new group, the American Association of Registered Nurses. This group will compete with the American Nurses Association in representing nurses at the national level.[20]

Shortages of Nurses

Since World War II, hospitals in the United States have coped with cyclical shortages of nurses. The shortages have generally been related to economic factors. When the overall economy declines, married nurses and working mothers, who represent a substantial portion of the workforce, are more likely to seek work or increase their hours; in better economic times they may be less likely to work or may only work part-time.[21] As in other fields, higher wages and better jobs encourage more nurses to seek employment.

In the 1990s, the growth of managed care slowed employment growth for registered nurses in hospitals, particularly in states such as California.[22,23] There was a surplus of registered nurses; some nurses lost their jobs, and some new nurses were unable to find jobs. Although hospitals were still hiring more registered nurses (Figure 1), it seemed that they might need fewer in the long term. Enrollment in nursing schools declined (Figure 3).

---

[17] Freudenheim & Villarosa.

[18] Rojas-Burke, J., & Lawton, W. Y. (2001, December 19). Staffing at heart of OHSU strike. *Oregonian.*

[19] Hirsch, B. T., & Macpherson, D. A. (2001). *Union membership and earnings data book: Compilations from the Current Population Survey.* Washington, DC: Bureau of National Affairs.

[20] Tieman, J. (2002). New nursing group divides ANA: AARN piggybacks on CNA's success, fights for nurse-staffing ratios. *Modern Healthcare, 32*(6), 13.

[21] AHA Commission.

[22] Buerhaus, P. I., & Staiger, D. O. (1996). Managed care and the nurse workforce. *Journal of the American Medical Association, 276*, 1487–1493.

[23] Buerhaus, P. I., & Staiger, D. O. (1999). Trouble in the nurse labor market? Recent trends and future outlook. *Health Affairs, 18*(1), 214–222.

Figure 3 Enrollment in Educational Programs to Train Registered Nurses in the United States

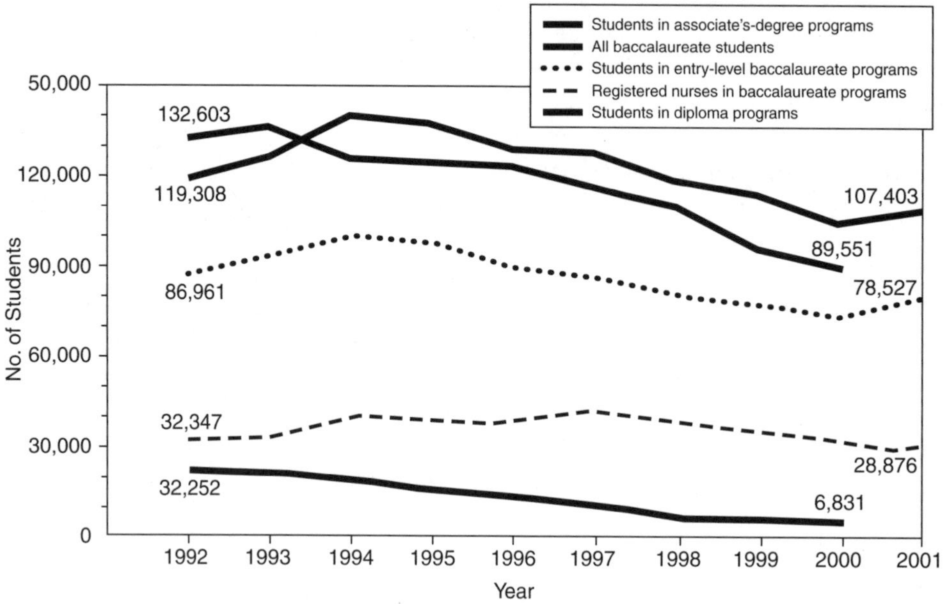

Source: Data for baccalaureate programs are from the American Association of Colleges of Nursing. Data for associate's-degree and diploma programs are from the National League for Nurisng.

Measuring the Shortages

Shortages of hospital nurses are sometimes difficult to evaluate.[24] Among the potential measures of a shortage are reports by hospital officials or nurses, the vacancy rate for nursing positions, the turnover rate for these positions, the number of nurses at a hospital after adjustment for the number of inpatients and the case mix, and the supply of registered nurses per 100,000 population. Although there is no gold standard, a recent study found the strongest relations between reports by hospital officials or nurses of a moderate or severe nursing shortage and job-vacancy rates.[24] Differences in the supply of nurses per capita did not predict which regions would have a majority of hospitals reporting shortages.

The number of employed registered nurses per capita varies widely from state to state (Figure 4). In 2000, the national average was 782 employed nurses per 100,000 population. California had only 544, whereas Massachusetts had 1,194 and Pennsylvania had 1010.[25] These variations have been cited as evidence of regional shortages of nurses, particularly in states with a low supply of nurses, such as California,[26] Nevada,[27] and Texas.[28] The demand for hospital-based nurses, however,

[24]Grumbach, K., Ash, M., Seago, J. A., Spetz, J., & Coffman, J. (2001). Measuring shortages of hospital nurses: How do you know a hospital with a nursing shortage when you see one? *Medical Care Research Review, 58*, 387–403.
[25]Spratley et al.
[26]Coffman, J., & Spetz, J. (1999). Maintaining an adequate supply of RNs in California. *Journal of Nursing Scholarship, 31*, 389–393.
[27]Richmond, E. (2002, January, 14). New hospitals face staffing woes: Nursing shortage is 'reaching crisis levels in Nevada.' *Las Vegas Sun*, 1.
[28]Miller, D. R. (2000, Winter). *Health and nurses in Texas: The supply of registered nurses: First look at available data, 1*(1). San Antonio: University of Texas Health Science Center.

reflects many factors, including the number of hospital beds, the average length of stay, the specific medical services offered, population growth, and the number of elderly residents. Although Florida has 785 nurses per 100,000 population—about the national average—the supply has been considered inadequate because the state has the highest percentage of elderly persons in the nation.[29] Because a low supply of nurses may reflect a low demand—not an unmet demand—for hospital-based nurses, the importance of the variations in and of themselves is uncertain.

Figure 4 Employed Registered Nurses per 100,000 Population

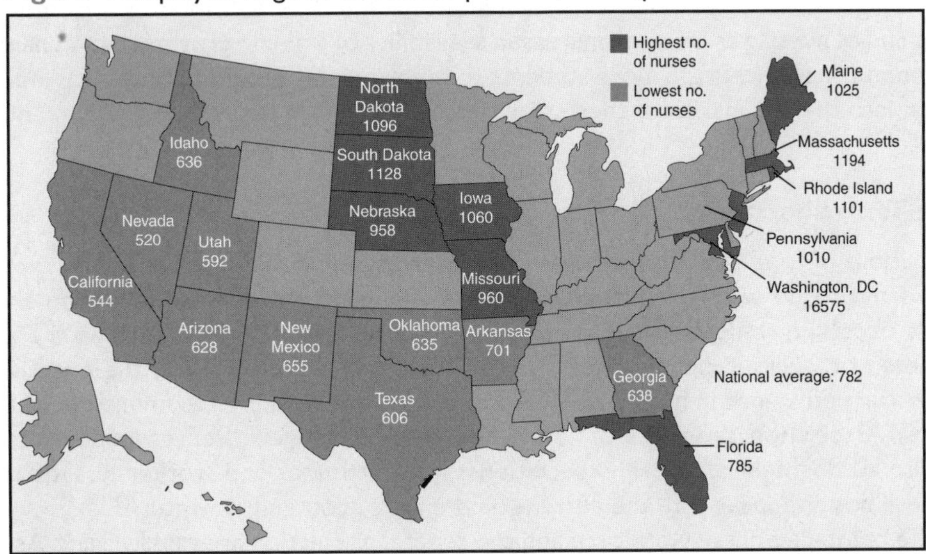

Note: Highest number of nurses is considered above average. Lowest number of nurses is considered below average. Although Florida has an average number of nurses (785) that is slightly above the national average of 782, it is included in the discussion in the article as a state that has a below-average number of nurses.
Source: Data are from the National Sample Survey of Registered Nurses, March 2000.

The Current Shortage

The current shortage of nurses began in 1998 in intensive care units and operating rooms.[30] It has since spread to labor-and-delivery units and general medical and surgical wards. The shortage is widespread throughout the country.

In 2001, the mean vacancy rate for registered-nurse positions at a given hospital was 13 percent. Fifteen percent of hospitals reported vacancy rates of 20 percent or more.[31] Mean vacancy rates were 11 percent in the Northeast and Midwest, 13 percent in the South, and 15 percent in the West. There were about 126,000 vacant positions nationwide.[32] Eighty-two percent of hospitals reported that it was more difficult to recruit registered nurses in 2001 than it had been in 1999; 1 percent said that it was less difficult.[33] According to a 2001 survey of chief executive officers of

---

[29] *Florida's nursing shortage: It is here and it is getting worse* (2001, November). Orlando: Florida Hospital Association.

[30] Buerhaus, P. I., Staiger, D. O., & Auerbach, D. I. (2000). Why are shortages of hospital RNs concentrated in speciality care units? *Nursing Economics, 18*, 1–6.

[31] *The healthcare workforce shortage and its implications for America's hospitals* (2001, Fall). Long Beach, CA.: First Consulting Group.

[32] *The hospital workforce shortage: Immediate and future* (2001, June). *TrendWatch, 3(2)*. Washington, DC: American Hospital Association, 1-8.

[33] *The healthcare workforce shortage.*

hospitals, 84 percent of hospitals had shortages of registered nurses; the next most frequently cited job categories with shortages were radiology and nuclear imaging (71 percent) and pharmacy (46 percent).[34] Of registered nurses working in nursing who were surveyed in 2001 and 2002, 95 percent thought there was a shortage of nurses, and 88 percent thought that the supply of registered nurses working in patient care in their community was lower than the demand.[35] National data about the current shortage of nurses are corroborated by reports from various states, including California,[36,37] Florida,[38] Maryland,[39] Nevada,[40] New York,[41] and Texas.[42]

The current shortage of nurses, albeit severe, may be similar to cyclical shortages that have occurred during the past 50 years. Better wages and better jobs, as well as better marketing of nursing schools and of nursing as a career, increased availability of training programs, and changes in the general economy, may encourage more students to enter nursing programs and bring more current nurses back into the job market. If these short-term factors are addressed, the current shortage should abate.

The Long-Term Shortage

Many predictions of long-term shortages or surpluses of physicians or other health care workers have turned out to be wrong. Nevertheless, there is the potential for a long-term shortage of nurses. This possibility reflects changing demographic and other factors, such as the decreased attractiveness of careers in health care to those entering employment and the dissatisfaction of people who currently work in hospitals.[43,44] According to the workforce commission of the American Hospital Association, shortages of nurses and other employees "reflect fundamental changes in population demographics, career expectations, work attitudes and worker dissatisfaction. The shortages will not disappear with the current or the next economic downturn."[45]

Both the registered-nurse workforce and the general population are rapidly aging. As members of the "baby boom" generation begin to retire, the demand for nurses is expected to increase rapidly.[46] Between 2000 and 2010, the occupation of registered nurse will be one of the five occupations with the greatest growth in the number of jobs, according to the Bureau of Labor Statistics. It is projected that during this period, there will be 1,000,400 job openings for registered nurses, including 561,000 new positions.[47]

---

[34]AHA Commission.

[35]*NurseWeek.*

[36]Coffman et al.

[37]Coffman & Spetz.

[38]Florida's nursing shortage.

[39]*Widespread hospital workforce shortages* (2001, June 26). Press release of the Association of Maryland Hospitals & Health Systems, Elkridge.

[40]Packham, J. F., & The Nevada Nurse Task Force (2001, March). *The nursing workforce and nursing education in Nevada.* Reno, NV: Nevada Hospital Association.

[41]Brewer, C. S., & Kovner, C. T. (2000). *A report on the supply and demand for registered nurses in New York State.* Latham, NY: New York State Nurses Association.

[42]Miller.

[43]Aiken et al.

[44]Levine, L. (2001, May 18). *A shortage of registered nurses: Is it on the horizon or already here?* Washington, DC: Congressional Research Service.

[45]AHA Commission.

[46]Buerhaus, P. I., Staiger, D. O., & Auerbach, D. I. (2000). Implications of an aging registered nurse workforce. *JAMA, 283,* 2948–2954.

[47]Hecker, D. E. (2001, November). Occupational employment projections to 2010. *Monthly Labor Review,* 57–84.

Younger nurses are more likely than older nurses to work in hospitals. In 2000, only 9 percent of registered nurses were less than 30 years of age, as compared with 25 percent in 1980 (Figure 5). About a third of registered nurses were 50 years of age or older.[48] A related issue is that nursing, particularly in a hospital, can be physically demanding and lead to occupational injuries, particularly for older nurses.[49] By 2020, a shortage of more than 400,000 registered nurses is possible.[50] One analysis concluded: "The evidence suggests a not-too-distant collision between the aging and shrinking RN workforce and the increasing demand driven (among other things) by the expanding population of Medicare beneficiaries."[51]

Figure 5 Age Distribution of Registered Nurses in the United States, 1980 through 2000

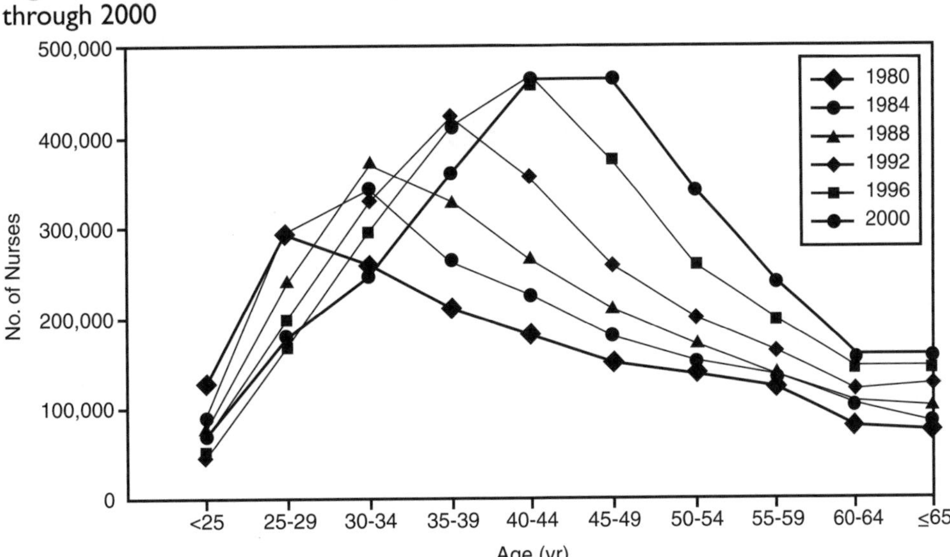

Source: Adapted from the National Sample Survey of Registered Nurses, March 2000.[48]

Minimal Nurse-Staffing Ratios

In 1999, the California legislature, prompted by concern about the effects of decreased levels of staffing by nurses on the quality of care, required the state Department of Health Services to establish minimal staffing ratios of nurses to patients according to the types of licensed-nurse classification and hospital unit.[52,53] In January 2002, Governor Gray Davis announced the proposed ratios (Table 1).[54] The actual regulations are likely to be finalized later this year, after public comments and hearings, and to take effect by July 2003.

48Spratley et al.

49Wunderlich et al.

50Buerhaus et al.

51Buerhaus, P. I., Staiger, D. O., & Auerbach, D. I. (2000). Policy responses to an aging registered nurse workforce. *Nursing Economics, 18*, 278–284, 303.

52State of California, Assembly Bill No. 394, Ch. 945 (Approved by Governor, October 19, 1999).

53Spetz, J., Seago, J. A., Coffman, J., Rosenoff, E., & O'Neill, E. (2000, December). Minimum nurse staffing ratios in California acute hospitals. Oakland: California Healthcare Foundation.

54Governor Gray Davis announces proposed nurse-to-patient ratios. Press release of the Office of the Governor of California, Sacramento, January 22, 2002.

The staffing ratios have been the subject of sharp disputes between the California Nurses Association, which worked for years to pass the legislation, and the California Healthcare Association, which represents hospitals in the state and has opposed the approach.[55] The nurses' association advocated a minimal ratio of 1 nurse to 3 patients on medical–surgical units; the hospital association advocated a minimal ratio of 1:10.

The proposed ratios include a minimum of one nurse to six patients on general medical–surgical units (Table 1). This minimum would change to one nurse to five patients 12 to 18 months after the regulations go into effect. Although most of the nurses are likely to be registered nurses, the extent to which licensed practical nurses could be substituted is not yet clear. For labor-and-delivery units, the minimal staffing ratio is one nurse to two patients. Intensive care units are already subject to a minimum of one nurse to two patients. The ratios are meant to be minimums; hospitals are expected to increase levels of staffing when patients require additional care.

Table 1 Proposed Minimal Nurse-Staffing Ratios for Hospital Units in California*

Hospital Unit	Proposed Ratio of Nurses to Patients
Intensive or critical care**	1:2
Neonatal intensive care**	1:2
Intermediate care nursery**	1:4
Labor and delivery	1:2
Postanesthesia care	1:2
Emergency department	
General	1:4***
Critical care	1:2
Trauma	1:1
Pediatrics	1:4
Step-down with telemetry	1:4
Specialty care (oncology)	1:5
General medical-surgical	1:6****
Behavioral health or psychiatric	1:6

*Data are staffing ratios proposed by the California Department of Health Services in January 2002 under Assembly Bill 394, which was signed into law in 1999. The actual regulations—which have yet to be finalized—are to take effect in 2003. Although most of the nurses are expected to be registered nurses, the proposed ratios do not specify when licensed practical nurses can be used. Not all types of hospital units are listed.

**Minimal nurse-to-patient ratios are already in place for these units by California statute, regulations, or both.

***Triage, radiology, or other specialty nurses are considered to represent an additional workforce; they are not included in this ratio.

****This ratio is an initial ratio; a ratio of 1:5 is to be phased in 12 to 18 months after the effective date of the regulations.

[55] DeMoro, R. (2002, January 31). New nurse-patient ratios will ensure better care. *Los Angeles Times*, B-19.

Complying with the Ratios

California has 470 hospitals, according to the California Healthcare Association. Fifteen percent of hospitals with medical–surgical units would not be in compliance with the initial ratio if it took effect now, and 36 percent would not be in compliance with the final ratio, according to Joanne Spetz of the Center for California Health Workforce Studies at the University of California, San Francisco.[56] Fifteen percent of hospitals with labor-and-delivery units would not be in compliance with the proposed ratio.

Spetz predicted that the cost of implementing the recommendations would be "rather small," because many hospitals would have to hire few, if any, additional nurses. She estimated the annual per-hospital increase in expenditures for nursing as $143,846 (1.0 percent) for the initial ratios and $217,210 (1.7 percent) for the final ratios.[57] The California Healthcare Association has not prepared per-hospital estimates. It has estimated that if 5,000 additional registered nurses are required statewide, the annual cost might be $400 million. It is possible, however, that the costs of hiring additional nurses may be offset if patients have fewer complications and adverse events and therefore leave the hospital sooner.

Reaction to the Ratios

According to Rose Ann DeMoro, the executive director of the California Nurses Association, minimal nurse-staffing ratios "are a dramatic step forward for hospitals in California" and will help to "create conditions in hospitals for nurses to return." Jan Emerson, vice president of external affairs at the California Healthcare Association, said that although "the hospital industry agrees with the notion that more nurses is probably a good thing," the minimal staffing ratios could have "serious unintended consequences." These include an inability to find qualified registered nurses, which may force hospitals to eliminate beds and reduce access to care. The proposed ratios also raise practical issues, such as whether the level of staffing is required around the clock.

The new American Association of Registered Nurses is encouraging other states to enact similar legislation. Mary Foley, the president of the American Nurses Association, said that her organization was "not opposed to the California bill but did not support it enthusiastically." She said that, although "10 to 12 patients per nurse is horrible," safe medical and nursing care is "not just a matter of numbers." Aiken, of the University of Pennsylvania School of Nursing, predicted that unless a "floor" for staffing is established, "we are not going to be able to stop the flight of nurses from hospitals. . . . If it is feasible to implement the ratios, a lot of other states may follow."

Mandatory Overtime

Some people like to work overtime, because they can make more money or take other time off. Others prefer to work on a regular schedule. Although it might seem inefficient and expensive for an employer to hire too few employees and then pay higher wages for overtime, this approach reduces the number of permanent employees and is one way to cope with vacancies.

Overtime has unique aspects in health care. Physicians and nurses have professional obligations to care for their patients and not abandon them. Although overtime is essential in emergencies, there is concern that hospitals, like other businesses, are using it instead to compensate for inadequate levels

---

[56] Spetz, J. (2002, January 24). *Revised cost estimates of minimum nurse-to-patient ratio proposals.* San Francisco: UCSF Center for Health Workforce Studies.

[57] Ibid.

of staffing. Exhausted nurses, like exhausted physicians, can pose safety risks. "By far the riskiest result of understaffing is the abuse of mandatory overtime as a staffing tool," Foley of the American Nurses Association stated in congressional testimony in March of this year.[58] Many nurses, she said, are being required to work some mandatory or unplanned overtime every month or face dismissal for insubordination or being reported to the state board of nursing for abandonment of patients.

In the recent national survey of working nurses,[59] 61 percent of respondents said they had observed increases in overtime or double shifts during the past year. Forty-eight percent said that "the amount of overtime required" had increased, 6 percent said it had decreased, and 45 percent said it had remained the same. Forty-five percent said working overtime was "strictly voluntary," 32 percent said it was "voluntary but feels like it is required," and 20 percent said it was "required" (Buerhaus, P., Vanderbilt University School of Nursing, personal communication). A national survey of oncology nurses, conducted in 2000, had similar findings (Buerhaus, P., personal communication).[60]

As of early May 2002, six states had enacted laws that ban or limit mandatory overtime, except in emergencies—Maine,[61] Maryland,[62] Minnesota,[63] Oregon,[64] New Jersey,[65] and Washington.[66] The Washington law prohibits hospitals from requiring nurses who care for patients from working more than 12 hours in a 24-hour period or more than 80 hours in a period of 14 consecutive days. Many of the other laws have similar provisions. More states are likely to enact such laws, which are backed by the American Nurses Association and other nursing organizations.

Potential Solutions

A major goal of minimal nurse-staffing ratios or the prohibition of mandatory overtime is to improve the quality of care. These measures may exacerbate shortages in the short term because hospitals will most likely have to hire more registered nurses. However, if they help to make hospitals more attractive places to work, they may make it easier to recruit nurses. Their actual effects will not be clear for at least several years.

The potential solutions to the shortage of nurses and related problems include expanding enrollment in nursing schools and bringing more men and members of minority groups into the profession.[67,68] They also include developing incentives to encourage nurses who work part-time to work more hours, offering better salaries, providing more regular work hours, and restructuring hospitals to make the work environment more attractive. In its recent report, the workforce commission of the American Hospital Association emphasized the need to make hospital work more meaningful and rewarding.[69] Still other approaches, such as recruiting more nurses from overseas[70] or encouraging affluent patients to hire their own nurses,[71] are less likely to have broad effects.

---

[58]Foley, M. (2002, March 7). *Statement for the Committee on Ways and Means, Subcommittee on Health regarding improving patient safety.* Washington, DC: American Nurses Association.

[59]NurseWeek.

[60]Buerhaus, P., Donelan, D., DesRoches, D., Lamkin, L., & Mallory, G. (2001). State of the oncology nursing workforce: Problems and implications for strengthening the future. *Nursing Economics, 19,* 198–208.

[61]Maine Pub. L. Ch. 401 (2001).

[62]Md. Senate bill 537, Ch. 322. Signed by the Governor May 6, 2002. Retrieved May 10, 2002, from http://mlis.state.md.us/2002rs/billfile/SB0537.htm.)

[63]Minnesota Mandatory Overtime Prevention Act, SF 2463/HF 2993, (2002).

[64]N.J. Pub. L. 2001, Ch. 300 (approved Jan. 2, 2002).

[65]Oregon HB 2800-B (effective Oct. 1, 2002).

[66]Washington, DC (2002), Senate Bill 6675/House Bill 2601.

[67]Coffman & Spetz.

[68]Buerhaus, et al.

[69]AHA Commission

[70]Brubaker, B. (2001, June 11). Hospitals go abroad to fill slots for nurses: Wide pay gap exists between U.S., foreign workers in D.C. area. *Washington Post,* A1.

[71]Zuger, A. (2002, April 16). Nurse deficit? Affluent patients hire their own. *New York Times* D1, D6.

Some combination of these approaches is likely to be most effective. Financial incentives may be particularly important. Many hospitals are paying nurses signing bonuses of $1,000 to $5,000 or more and are temporarily filling vacant positions with registry or traveling nurses.[72,73] In Boston, Tufts–New England Medical Center has agreed to raise nurses' pay 18 to 23 percent over a period of 23 months.[74] Nurses at the Oregon Health and Science University will receive at least a 20 percent raise over a three-year period.[75]

The American Nurses Credentialing Center, a subsidiary of the American Nurses Association, has developed the "magnet nursing services recognition program" for hospitals that meet quality standards and provide nurses with more responsibilities, autonomy, and opportunities to participate in policy decisions. Studies suggest that nurses in such hospitals have greater job satisfaction, and the hospitals are less likely to have difficulty hiring and retaining nurses.[76] As part of the new contract for nurses, the Oregon Health and Science University agreed to seek "magnet" status.

Enrollment in associate's-degree programs for nurses decreased through 2000, according to preliminary data (Figure 3). One encouraging sign, however, is that enrollment in baccalaureate programs, which appeal to younger students,[77] has increased[78] (Figure 3). The increase—in 2001—ended a six-year period of declining enrollment. The Nurse Reinvestment Act would authorize federal funding for scholarships and loan repayments for nurses who agree to work after graduation in areas where there are shortages, as well as for public-service announcements that would promote nursing as a career.[79] The Bush administration has announced the availability of grants and has proposed extending loan-repayment programs.[80] In California, Governor Davis has proposed a $60 million initiative for the nurse workforce that expands training programs for nurses.[81]

The Future

Nurses who work in hospitals are apprehensive about the future. Hospitals employ many more registered nurses than physicians and cannot function without them. At a time of serious financial constraints, however, they must often choose between hiring more nurses and launching or maintaining other programs that may improve patient care, such as computerized order-entry systems.[82] Some of the issues raised by nurses about hospital staffing reflect their interest in their own financial and job security. Yet there is ample evidence of a broader unease.

Many tensions will be difficult, if not impossible, to resolve, particularly if additional funds do not become available. For example, within the nursing profession, higher-quality care may mean a

---

[72]NurseWeek.

[73]*The healthcare workforce shortage.*

[74]Barnard.

[75]Rojas-Burke J., & Lawton, W. Y. (2002, February 7). OHSU, nurses reach a deal. *Oregonian*, A1.

[76]Aiken, L. H. (in press). Superior outcomes for magnet hospitals: The evidence base. In McClure, M. L., & Hinshaw, A. S. (Eds.), *Magnet hospitals revisited: Attraction and retention of professional nurses.* Washington DC: American Nurses Publishing.

[77]Auerbach, D. I., Buerhaus, P. I., & Staiger, D. O. (2000). Associate degree graduates and the rapidly aging RN workforce. *Nursing Economics, 18*, 178–184.

[78]*Enrollments rise at U.S. nursing colleges and universities ending a six-year period of decline* (2001, December 20). Press release of the American Association of Colleges of Nursing, Washington, DC.

[79]*Nurse Reinvestment Act* (2001). H.R. 3487, par. 1864.

[80]*Bush administration promotes careers in nursing* (2002, February 22). Press release of the Department of Health and Human Services, Washington, DC.

[81]*Governor Davis announces nurse workforce initiative* (2002, January 23). Press release of the Office of the Governor of California, Sacramento.

[82]Landro, L. (2002, March 15). Deadly hospital errors prompt group to push for technological help. *Wall Street Journal*, B1.

better-educated workforce, with a higher percentage of nurses with bachelor's or advanced degrees. Such a workforce, however, would expect more responsibility and greater independence and would be more expensive to hire and retain.

In the long term, the future of the nursing profession is related to its ability to attract more young nurses, to support the careers of current nurses, and to create more jobs for nurses with higher wages and greater responsibilities. Such efforts can be successful only if the positions students are training to fill are sufficiently attractive, as compared with the alternatives in other fields. "Nursing is a worthy career," said Foley, the president of the American Nurses Association. "It should not be considered secondary or inferior. We want nursing back on the list of career choices for bright young men and women who are looking at health care."

Activity: Vocabulary Development

Reading 2.3 contains many medical/nursing terms and socio-economic terms that are used to describe the current crisis in nursing. Add the words you do not know to your dictionary, following the guidelines on page 33. Use a medical English dictionary to look up the medical/nursing terms and a college-level English dictionary to look up the socio-economic terms that you do not know. Use 10–15 new words in answering the discussion questions.

Comprehension and Discussion Questions

Read through the entire article and answer the questions. These questions will help you to compare and contrast information provided in the three readings, as well as the different perspectives of the authors.

1. What did Needleman and colleagues discover about the relationship between nursing care and patient outcomes? Why are the findings of this study significant in a discussion of nursing, especially within the context of a nursing crisis? Compare the discussion of these findings to Gordon's perspective on the topic of "failure to rescue" (page 51) in Reading 2.2 (See Question 3.)
2. Based on Figure 1 on page 67, "between 1983 and 2000, the staffing levels of registered nurses in hospitals increased by 37 percent" (page 66). What is Gordon's perspective in Reading 2.2 on the hospital claim that there has been an increase in the number of nurses working in hospitals? What are "case managers" or "utilization reviewers" (page 47)? How do their responsibilities differ from those who provide direct care?
3. Based on Figure 1, "the ratio of registered nurses to hospitalized patients remained relatively constant between 1994 and 2000" (page 66). Is this finding consistent with Gordon's perspective in Reading 2.2 on the increase in patient load? (See Question 1.) Why do you think Steinbrook and Gordon have different perspectives on this issue?
4. Steinbrook writes: "The *perception* is that physicians and hospital administrators often treat registered nurses as workers, not as clinicians and peers, and when possible seek to replace them with less skilled and cheaper per-

sonnel, such as licensed practical nurses and aides" (page 68). What is the effect of the word perception in the above quote? What data does Steinbrook provide in his discussion on nurse dissatisfaction? How is Steinbrook's discussion different in tone from Gordon's discussion of nurse dissatisfaction in Reading 2.2? (See Questions 1 and 2.)

5. What was the average annual salary of nurses in 2000? (See Figure 2 on page 68.) Gordon claims in "What Nurses Stand For" that "nursing does provide attractive middle-income salaries" (1997, 84). Based on the information in Figure 2, would Steinbrook agree with Gordon? Why or why not?
6. What reasons are given for the shortage of nurses that began in the 1990s? How do these reasons compare with the discussion of the nursing shortage in Reading 2.1 (see Question 1) and Reading 2.2 (see Question 5)?
7. What are cyclical shortages, and what causes them? According to Steinbrook, how is the current shortage of nurses similar to cyclical shortages of nurses in the past?
8. Is Steinbrook convinced that a long-term shortage is inevitable? What words or phrases does the author use on pages 72–73 to indicate his opinion about this topic?
9. What are possible short-term and long-term effects on the nursing shortage of establishing minimal nurse-staffing ratios and banning or limiting mandatory overtime?
10. The author writes that "higher-quality care may mean a better-educated workforce, with a higher percentage of nurses with bachelor's or advanced degrees. Such a workforce, *however,* would expect more responsibility and greater independence and would be more expensive to hire and retain" (pages 77–78)? What is the effect of the word *however* in this quote? Why is the author concerned? Is the author sympathetic, do you think, to the plight of nurses today? Why or why not? Provide support for your answer.

Writing about Nursing: Analyzing and Applying Information

Now that you have read and discussed contemporary issues in nursing, choose Question 1 and either Question 2, 3, or 4 and write a two- to three-page essay in response to the questions. Use information from the readings in this chapter, as well as from your own personal experiences with the health care system, to develop and support your points.

1. Why is there a nursing shortage?
2. How has the nursing shortage affected the profession of nursing?
3. What solutions would you propose for solving the nursing shortage?
4. In your opinion, is it a difficult time to be going into nursing, or a time of opportunity, both in general and for you personally?

UNIT 3

Writing about Culture in Nursing

The **content-based objectives** include understanding the role of culture in terms of

- The perception of and response to health and illness
- Patients' responses to pain
- Nursing practice
- Pain management

The **skill-based objectives** include

- Locating books and articles on nursing and health care, using online library catalogs and nursing/allied health databases
- Incorporating information from outside sources through paraphrasing and quoting
- Documenting use of outside sources through in-text citations and reference list
- Integrating information from outside sources through introductory sentences and verb choice
- Writing a summary and critique of a nursing research article
- Writing a research paper on cultural influences on nursing practice

At the end of the unit, you will reflect on the cultural influences in your life and their influence on your future practice as a nurse.

Writing is an essential skill in nursing education, used to both help you understand as well as demonstrate your understanding of nursing content. Knowledge about culture and the role of culture in health care is an essential component of nursing in the 21st century. Nurses need to understand how culture, in particular cultural values, beliefs, attitudes, and practices, influence their clients' as well as their own perceptions and responses to health and illness. This unit begins with writing as a means to explore the role of culture in nursing. By writing about culture in nursing, you will both practice an essential language skill and learn about essential content in nursing education.

Writing in Nursing

In nursing programs, there are essentially two different contexts for writing: in the classroom and in the clinical setting.

Writing in the Nursing Classroom

As part of your coursework, you will complete written assignments of various kinds, such as analyses of client assessments, nursing care plans, reflections on clinical experiences, and traditional research papers. You may also be asked to write personal philosophy papers, teaching-learning plans, and clinical preparation papers.

For papers that require use of secondary sources, such as traditional research papers, you will need to locate appropriate sources of information and evaluate their credibility. In addition, you will need to integrate information from outside sources into your own writing, using research-based writing skills, such as paraphrasing, quoting, and citing sources. You will also need to analyze, synthesize, and apply information in some way that goes beyond simply reporting it. You will also need to distinguish between factual information and an author's assertions, interpretations, and opinions, especially in articles that report research findings.

In many ways the research papers that you write in nursing courses are not that different from papers you may have written for college writing classes. Although the content is about nursing and related issues, some strategies and techniques you learned in college writing classes will apply to writing papers in nursing programs.

On the other hand, there are discipline-specific skills in writing in nursing that are not the same as general academic writing. For example, a personal perspective is generally not accepted in nursing courses, other than for personal reflective papers and personal journals about clinical experiences. In addition, because of and in preparation for the need to be brief and precise in meaning when making patient progress notes in the clinical setting, writing in nursing coursework also tends to favor brevity and precision.

Writing in the Clinical Setting

In the clinical setting, nursing students write notes about patient progress also referred to as charting. In progress notes, students document their assessment of clients and the treatments they administer.

Nursing students also prepare for clinical work by writing a proposed nursing care plan for patients to whom they are assigned. Proposed care plans must reflect a thorough understanding of the patient's diagnosis, as well as prescribed medications and treatments, and must be supported by evidence and relevant theory. These plans—which parallel the nursing process of assessing, diagnosing, planning, implementing, intervention, and evaluation—help students learn to think critically about nursing practice.

Locating Information from Outside Sources

For traditional research papers in nursing and for nursing care plans, you will need to locate and integrate information from outside sources. In this chapter, you will be assigned to write a paper on culture and nursing, using information from outside sources. In addition to support your points, you will need to provide specific examples from different cultural communities.

Outside sources are usually written sources, but they can also be oral sources. If you are asked to conduct original research, you may need to interview experts in the field or even clients. In such cases, the people you interview are referred to as oral sources.

Primary and Secondary Sources

Another important distinction of sources is between primary and secondary sources. **Primary sources** are original materials, such as news reports and government statistics. They are also first-hand materials or personal materials written by someone, like diaries and letters, memoirs and autobiographies. Information that is gathered directly from individuals, through interviews and questionnaires, is also considered primary. For your own research study, when you interview people or gather information through surveys or questionnaires, you are gathering **primary data.** Indeed, your own research study, for which you gather your own data, is called **primary research.**

Secondary sources, on the other hand, are works that analyze or comment on primary materials. They are one step removed from the original source. For example, books that analyze and interpret historical events or articles that report on research studies are secondary sources. Research papers in nursing are usually based on written, secondary sources unless students are specifically asked to design and implement their own research study or to incorporate primary sources into their research papers, such as government health statistics or primary data, such as the results of interviews with clients.

Finding Books Using Online Library Catalogs

Online catalogs list a library's own collection, as well as collections available from other libraries. You can often request books and materials from affiliated libraries to be sent to your home library for pick-up. Books that are not available in your library or from affiliated libraries can be requested through Interlibrary Loan (ILL).

Requesting a book through ILL is easy to do; most libraries have the request form online. Simply fill out the form and submit it. Your library will send the request to a library that has a copy of the book you want. A staff member at that library will retrieve the book and send it to your library, where you can pick it up and then use for a limited period of time, usually three weeks, at no charge or for a minimal fee.

If you are requesting an article through ILL, your request will be sent to a library that has a copy of the journal. A staff member at that library will retrieve the journal, make a copy of the article, and send it to your library. Your library will then send the article to you at the address you specified on the request form, again at no charge or for a minimal fee. Alternately, an electronic copy of the article may be sent to you at your email address. Either way, the process is easy and the result is the same: You get a copy of the article. It can take a week or so for a request to be filled through ILL, so plan ahead for the extra time needed.

To locate books on culture and nursing, use a **keyword** search. A keyword search identifies books with a particular word in its title or in the bibliographic information about the book that is stored in the online catalog.

For books on nursing and culture, combine keywords, such as *nursing* (or *health care*) and *culture* (or *cultural diversity* or *cultural competence* or *transcultural nursing*). For books on a particular cultural group and health care, combine keywords, such as *Hispanic Americans* and *health care.* In one library system, 22 books were located using this combination of keywords.

You could also try a **subject** search, but keyword searches usually result in more hits, or sources. Also, for subject searches, you need to know the Library of Congress subject headings that are used to classify material in libraries. Ask a reference librarian for help if you'd like to try a subject search. (Note that *health care* is not a Library of Congress subject heading.)

Locate two or three books that you could use for a research paper on culture and nursing. Try a keyword search.

List all the keywords that you tried. ________________________________

____

Which ones were the most productive? ____________________________

Explain your **Search History** (i.e., the various keywords and/or combinations of keywords you tried), and show a copy of your **Search Results** to your instructor.

Using Nursing Journal Databases

The largest online nursing journal database is **CINAHL,** which stands for *Cumulative Index to Nursing & Allied Health Literature.* Other databases that include nursing and allied health journals are **HealthSource** and **Alt-Health Watch.** Links to these and other health-related databases should be available through your library's homepage. Your library's reference desk may have handouts that provide you with steps for using these databases on campus, as well as how to access and use them off campus. The interface of these databases is constantly changing, so make sure you have the most current handouts.

Search your library's home page and/or talk with a reference librarian to answer these questions.

1. What nursing or health care databases do you have access to through your library?
2. What are the unique features of each of these databases?
3. Are there any handouts about specific resources or reference materials for nursing? If so, what are they? Obtain a copy of any handouts, and share them with your classmates.

Later in this chapter, you will be asked to summarize and critique an article about the health care experiences of an immigrant group in the United States. Begin your search for an appropriate article by looking in CINAHL.

Articles in CINAHL are organized using subject headings or descriptor terms (College of St. Catherine Libraries, 2004, 2006). Begin your search using these terms: *health beliefs, health behavior, attitude to health,* and *cultural values.*

To narrow your search, use *and* to combine these terms with appropriate terms for a particular cultural community. Link any alternate search terms with *or* and put them in parentheses. For example:

Hmong **and** *health beliefs*
(Hispanic Americans **or** *Latinos)* **and** *health behavior*
Ethiopians **and** *(health beliefs* **or** *health behavior)*

Using *and* has a ***restrictive*** or ***limiting*** effect on your search. In the first example, your search will access only articles that address **both** Hmong and health beliefs, not one or the other.

Using *or* has an ***expansive or broadening*** effect on your search. In the second example, your search will access articles that address either Hispanic Americans or Latinos and health behavior, and in the third example, Ethiopians and either health beliefs or health behavior.

Search Strategies

Some basic principles for combining search terms when you are finding too little are:

1. Use **more synonyms** as alternate search terms because more terms connected with *or* equals more hits:

   Hispanic **or** *Hispanics* **or** *Hispanic Americans* **or** *Latinos*

2. Use **more general terms** to search more broadly:

   Hispanics **rather than** *Hispanic Americans*
   health **rather than** *health beliefs* **or** *health behavior*

3. Use **fewer unrelated terms** connected with *and* because more terms connected with *and* equals fewer hits:

   Hispanic **and** *health*
   rather than
   Hispanic **and** *elderly* **and** *diseases* **and** *health beliefs*

Some basic principles for combining search terms when you are finding too much are:

1. Use **fewer synonyms** as alternate search terms because more terms connected with *or* equals more hits:

   Hispanic Americans **and** *health beliefs*
   rather than
   (Hispanic **or** *Hispanic Americans)* **and** *(health behaviors* **or** *health beliefs)*

2. Use **more specific terms** to search less broadly:

   Hispanic Americans **and** *health beliefs*
   rather than
   Hispanics **and** *health*

3. Use **more unrelated terms** connected with *and* because more terms connected with *and* equals fewer hits:

   Hispanic Americans **and** *diseases* **and** *elderly* **and** *health beliefs*
   rather than
   Hispanic Americans **and** *health beliefs*

Different combinations of keywords will result in different lists. In one library system, the more restricted (*Hispanic Americans* **and** *health beliefs*) yielded only three articles, but the more expansive (*Hispanic Americans* **or** *Latinos*) and (*health beliefs* **or** *health behavior* **or** *attitude to health* **or** *cultural values*) yielded 57.

Understanding the Results of Your Search

If you have done your search correctly, the result should be a list of articles that match your combination of descriptor terms, referred to as the Search Results. For each article listed in the Search Results, you should be able to access a citation and an abstract. The full text may also be available online; if not, the citation gives you all the information you need for locating the article in the library or for ordering it through Interlibrary Loan.

The **abstract** provides you with a brief, usually one-paragraph, summary of the article. For a research article, an abstract should include the focus or purpose of the research study, the methodology used, the results of the study, and implications for nursing practice. By reading the abstract, you should be able to tell if the article meets the criteria for an assignment.

A list of **citations** or **cited references** may also be part of the search results. This is a list at the end of an article of all the outside sources referred to in the article itself. This list can be helpful in locating additional books and articles that were not included in your Search Results.

Finding Other Online Sources

In addition to online nursing and other health care databases, there are many websites on the Internet related to nursing, medicine, or health care in general. A few are listed.

Nursing

www.nursingknowledge.org
Nursing Knowledge International—a non-profit organization that seeks to help nurses worldwide.

www.nurse.com
News and information for nurses and nursing students.

www.minoritynurse.com
Career and educational resources for minority nursing professionals, students, and faculty.

www.ninr.nih.gov/
National Institute of Nursing Research

Medicine Plus®

http://medlineplus.gov/
Service of National Library of Medicine and National Institute of Health—health topics, medical encyclopedia and dictionary, health news.

Health Care

http://ethnomed.org
Good source of information on culture and health care.

http://culturemed.sunyit.edu
Good source of information on culture and health care.

www.ihi.org/IHI/Topics
Institute for Healthcare Improvement

Evaluating Information from Websites

For sources available on the Internet, make sure the author is from a reputable health care organization or educational institution. Also, make sure the point of view expressed by the author is based on research that is balanced and supported by evidence.

Pages from .gov and .edu addresses are the most reliable sources on the Internet because the information has probably gone through a review process, based on established criteria. The websites are also likely to be well maintained and updated regularly. Nonprofit organizations, such as nursing associations, use an .org address and usually contain interesting, but general information.

Information that has been put on the Internet by commercial organizations or individuals has a .com address. Sources at .com addresses should be scrutinized carefully. Make sure that any information you use from the Internet, especially from individual websites, has been written by responsible practitioners or scholars in the field of nursing. Always check the credentials of the author or organization connected with the website. Look for this information on the home page, as well as on links to the home page. Do a Google™ search, using the author's name as the search term, and see what comes up. Check the author's credentials—educational background, current and former positions, and publications (especially books and articles in scholarly journals)—to make sure they are experts in their field.

Despite the need to be cautious with information from websites, information from the Internet is often much more up to date than information that has taken several years to be published in a journal or book. Whenever you have questions about an article or other information available online, ask your instructor to look at it, or ask a reference librarian to help you.

Integrating Information from Outside Sources

There are two ways to integrate information from outside sources into your own paper: paraphrasing or quoting. To **paraphrase** means to put something into your own words. To **quote** means to copy something word for word from its source. When you quote, you must put the words you have copied into **quotation marks.** Whether you quote or paraphrase information from an outside source, you must document the source by providing a **citation.**

Examples

Paraphrase Followed by Citation

Nurses from cultures that value self-control may misunderstand if patients from other ethnic groups express their emotions when they experience pain (Calvillo & Flaskerud, 1991).

Quote Followed by Citation

Another common stereotype is that "Mexican Americans have a low pain tolerance" (Cavillo & Flaskerud, 1991, p. 137).

Whether you paraphrase or quote, you must cite the outside source. You must also change more than a word or two when you paraphrase to avoid **unintentional plagiarism.** In addition to the words, you must also change the structure of the sentence. **Plagiarism** is a serious offense in U.S. academic culture. It occurs when the words students use in a paraphrase are too close to or are the same as words from the original source, even when the source has been cited. (See pages 95–96 for further discussion of plagiarism.)

Paraphrasing

Look at the example of original material, and then compare the plagiarized and paraphrased versions that follow. In the plagiarized version, the structure of the sentences is the same as in the original and only a few words have been changed. The words that have been changed or added are in italics.

Original

> Nursing candidates must prepare by a rigorous course of training that includes a thorough grounding in anatomy, physiology, pharmacology, the cause and treatment of disease, the intricacies of nutrition and diet, surgical skills, and a variety of techniques pertaining to patient care. Many nurses also prepare for more specialized work, such as the care of newborn infants, maternity patients, or the mentally ill, or for duties in the operating room. (HighBeam Encyclopedia, 2006, para. 2)

Plagiarized

> Nursing candidates must *also* prepare by rigorous courses *in school which* includes anatomy, physiology, pharmacology, the cause and treatment of a disease, the *importance* of nutrition and diet, surgical skills, and a variety of techniques *relating* to patient care. Many nurses also prepare for *a particular area of nursing*, such as the care of a newborn, maternity patients, the mentally ill, or for duties in the operating room.

Paraphrased

> Training to become a nurse includes mastery of many subjects, including: anatomy and physiology, pathophysiology or the study of diseases, pharmacology, nutrition, and the care and treatment of patients. In addition to general practice, many nurses decide to specialize in a particular area of patient care, such as care of maternity patients, newborns, children, the elderly, or the mentally ill, or a particular setting, such as the emergency room or the operating room.

The easiest way to avoid plagiarizing is to read the original many times until you understand it completely. Then, close the book or put the article away and write your understanding of the idea, focusing on its meaning, not the actual words used.

Activity: Paraphrasing

Read the quote and then paraphrase it. Do not begin in the same way as the original. Change the structure of the sentences, as well as most of the words.

Original

> Training for a career as a registered nurse (RN) can be met by several means: a two-year course at a junior college or a four-year degree program at a college or university. (Three-year courses given by hospitals are being phased out because of high costs.) Emphasis on college education for nurses is on the upsurge, because greater knowledge is required to apply the latest methods of diagnosis and therapy. Training includes both classroom study and actual hospital practice, and the graduate must still be examined and licensed by the state. (HighBeam Encyclopedia, 2006, para. 3)

Quoting

If you are unable to put something into your own words, either because it is too complicated or too technical, or because it would lose its effectiveness, you can **quote** it, by copying it word for word from the original and putting it in **quotation marks.**

Quoting Definitions

Definitions of common words from a dictionary do not need to be quoted, but definitions of specialized terms are best quoted, as in the following examples.

Examples

The American Nurses Association defines nursing as “the diagnosis and treatment of human responses to actual or potential health problems” (ANA, 1980, p. 9).

Culture is defined as “the non physical traits, such as values, beliefs, attitudes, and customs that are shared by a group of people and passed from one generation to the next” (Kozier, Erb, Berman, & Snyder, 2004b, p. 206).

Integrating Quotes

If the quote is not a complete sentence grammatically, you need to integrate it into your own writing by attaching it to one of your own sentences. In the previous example, "the diagnosis and treatment of human responses to actual or potential health problems" is a noun phrase; it is not a complete sentence as there is no subject or verb. The rest of the sentence, beginning with *the American Nurses Association,* completes the sentence grammatically.

If your quote is a complete sentence, and you just need to add an introductory phrase to provide a context for the quote, you still need to make sure that the grammar of the sentence works. The source (or author) of the quote should be included as the subject of the sentence, and the main verb should indicate the position or attitude of the author toward the quote.

Example

Calvillo and Flaskerud (1991) *indicate* that many Hispanics believe "one's fate is to suffer in this world" (p. 113).

In this example, the subject of the sentence is *Calvillo and Flaskerud,* the source of the quote, and the main verb is *indicate.* A noun clause, beginning with *that,* completes the sentence and connects the introductory phrase to the quoted material.

Using Quotes

Including too many quotes suggests in your paper that you have not really understood the ideas in your paper. It gives the impression that you have simply cut-and-pasted quotes to put together the paper, rather than used the more challenging skills of paraphrasing, analyzing, and synthesizing information from outside sources. A good rule to follow is: *Quote only what you cannot paraphrase.*

Sometimes there are specific reasons for using a quote, as in the following activity. In Reading 3.1, "Culture and Heritage" (Kozier et al., 2004b), there is only one quote. Look at the excerpt beginning on page 107. Locate the quote, and answer the questions.

1. How does the quote begin? ________________________
2. Is the quote a complete sentence? ________________________
3. Have the authors integrated the quote into their own sentence? _______

   If so, what is the subject of the sentence? ________________

   Main verb? ________________________________
4. Why have the authors introduced the quote in this way? ____________

   ____
5. What is the source of this quote? ________________________
6. Why, do you think, have the authors quoted this statement, rather than paraphrased it? ________________________

Adding or Substituting Words

When you integrate a quote into your own writing, sometimes you need to add words or otherwise make changes in the quote to clarify the meaning of a word or to make the grammar work. For example, a quote that includes a pronoun and not the original noun or noun phrase will not be clear. Or, a quote that refers to someone whose identity is not explained in the quote will not be clear. Such additions or substitutions are put inside **brackets** to show they are not part of the original quote.

Example

Even when the nurse was directing her questions at Mrs. Chen, Mrs. Chen "stares first at nurse, then at husband" (Herberg, 2003, p. 3). Mr. Chen would then answer for Mrs. Chen. After treating the Chens, "**[the nurse]** cannot understand why Mrs. Chen gave Phillip **[Chen's son]** cold tea nor why it took so long for the Chens to answer her simple question" (pp. 3–4).

In this example, the pronoun *she* has been replaced with the noun phrase *the nurse*, so the reader will know who *she* refers to. In addition, *Chen's son* has been added after *Phillip* to explain who he is.

Deleting Words

Only include in a quote the words that you need to make your point or complete your idea, even if that means eliminating words from the original text. Use **ellipsis** (or three dots) to indicate that words have been omitted from the quote, even if only one or two words have been eliminated.

> Example
>
> According to *Dorland's Illustrated Medical Dictionary* (2000), nursing is "the provision . . . of services that are essential to or helpful in the promotion, maintenance, and restoration of health and well-being or in the prevention of illness. . . ." (p. 1,248).

The complete text has been provided below for this quote. Read the complete text and compare it with the example. Then, answer the questions that follow.

> Nursing is "the provision, at various levels of preparation, of services that are essential to or helpful in the promotion, maintenance, and restoration of heath and well-being or in the prevention of illness, as of infants, of the sick and injured, or of others for any reason unable to provide such services for themselves. Sometimes designated according to the age of the patients being cared for (e.g., pediatric or geriatric nursing), or the particular health problems (e g., gynecologic, medical, obstetrical, orthopedic, psychiatric, surgical, urological nursing, or the like), or the setting in which the services are provided (e.g., office, school, or occupational health nurse)" (p. 1,248).

1. Cross out the words in the complete text that were not included in the example.
2. Why do you think the words you crossed out were not included in the example?

Documenting Outside Sources

Whether you paraphrase or quote something from an outside source, you must document your source, both within the paper itself and at the end of the paper, to avoid plagiarism. **Plagiarism** is a serious offense in U.S. academic culture. It occurs when students do not cite the source for ideas in their paper that are not theirs. (See pages 95–96 for further discussion of plagiarism.) **In-text citations** provide documentation within the paper. A **reference list** provides documentation at the end of the paper and includes all the outside sources you cited in your paper.

The format that is used in nursing to document outside sources follows conventions established by the American Psychological Association (APA). A complete description of this documentation system and all of its rules can be found in the *Publication Manual of the American Psychological Association*, available in the reference section of your library. You can also find information at the APA website: www.apastyle.org.

In-Text Citations

In APA, the in-text citation includes the last names of the author(s) and the date of publication, provided in parentheses after the paraphrased idea or quote. For quotes, the page number is also provided.

Examples

For a Paraphrase

Nurses from cultures that value self-control may misunderstand if patients from other ethnic groups express their emotions when they experience pain (Calvillo & Flaskerud, 1991).

For a Quote

Another common stereotype is that "Mexican Americans have a low pain tolerance" (Cavillo & Flaskerud, 1991, p. 137).

If you include the author's name(s) in the introductory phrase of the sentence, the author's last name(s) is not be included in the in-text citation. You would include just the date, and with quotes, also the page number, as in the following examples:

Examples

For a Paraphrase

As discussed by Calvillo and Flaskerud (1991), nurses from cultures that value self-control may misunderstand if patients from other ethnic groups express their emotions when they experience pain.

For a Quote

According to Calvillo and Flaskerud (1991), another common stereotype is that "Mexican Americans have a low pain tolerance" (p. 137).

Note that for a quote, you need to provide the date right after you refer to the author(s) and the page number at the end of the quote, as shown.

If you include information from interviews in your paper, you still need to provide an in-text citation. Include the last name of the person interviewed, the words "personal communication," and the year of the interview in parentheses, as in the following example:

Example

In 1992, the number of Hmong-American students at the post-secondary level in both Minnesota and Wisconsin was estimated to be 600 (Yang, personal communication, 1992).

Reference List

At the end of your paper, you need to provide a complete list of the works you cited in your paper. Use a writer's handbook or the APA publication manual to make sure you follow the correct format for the **reference list.**

In the example that follows, note these characteristics:

1. The reference list begins on a separate page. The title of the page is References. The title is centered, but no punctuation or additional formatting is added.
2. The list of works is alphabetized by the last names of the first author listed. The list is double-spaced throughout. For each listing, the first line begins at the left margin, the second and third lines are indented by half an inch.
3. For titles of books and articles, only the first word of each title and the first word after a colon are capitalized. Proper nouns and adjectives are also capitalized. In addition, titles of journals are capitalized, except for articles *(a, an),* coordinating conjunctions *(and, but, or, nor, so, for, and yet),* the *to* in an infinitive, and prepositions, unless they begin or end a title or subtitle.

In this reference list, the first item is an article published in a journal, the second is a book, and the third is a chapter from an anthology.

References

Calvillo, E. R., & Flaskerud, J. H. (1991). Review of literature on culture and pain of adults with focus on Mexican-Americans. *Journal of Transcultural Nursing 2,* 16–23.

Giger, J. N., & Davidhizar, R. E. (1999) *Transcultural nursing: Assessment and intervention.* (3rd ed.). St. Louis, MO: Mosby.

Herberg, P. (2003). Theoretical foundations of transcultural nursing. In J. S. Boyle & M. M. Andrews (Eds.), *Transcultural concepts in nursing care* (pp. 3–65). Philadelphia: Lippincott Williams & Wilkins.

Plagiarism from a Cultural Perspective

Plagiarism is defined in the *Longman Advanced American Dictionary* as: "to take words, ideas, etc., from someone else's work and use them in your work, without stating where they came from . . . as if they were your own ideas." Plagiarism occurs when students do not cite the source for ideas in their paper that are not theirs. Plagiarism also occurs when the words students use in a paraphrase are too close to or are even the same as words from the outside source even when the source has been cited.

International students and recent immigrants sometimes plagiarize because they are not aware it is considered a serious offense in U.S. academic culture. They may be unfamiliar with the American concept of individuals owning ideas and the value placed on original thinking. Indeed, in some cultures, students are expected to memorize the ideas of the masters and to use the original wording of these ideas in their own writing as a sign of respect for the authority of those ideas.

Students also plagiarize because they have not yet developed the skill of paraphrasing or because they lack the confidence in their ability to paraphrase well. No doubt paraphrasing is a complicated skill, but it can be learned! If you don't think you can effectively paraphrase what the author said, then use quotation marks or talk to your teacher about how to paraphrase and summarize what someone else has said.

In small groups, answer these questions about the use of outside sources.

1. How does your native culture view using outside sources in writing assignments?
2. Are there rules you must follow when you use outside sources? If so, what are they?
3. Are there rules you must follow to document your outside sources? If so, what are they?
4. Have you ever been accused of plagiarizing? What happened? What would you do differently in that situation today? Why?
5. What concerns do you have about rules and conventions in the United States regarding the use and documentation of outside sources?

Referring to Outside Sources

There are many ways to integrate information from outside sources into your paper. In a summary, for example, you need to introduce the article you are summarizing in the first or introductory sentence.

Introducing the Article and Author(s)

In the introductory sentence, include the title of the article, the author(s), and the date of publication. See the examples for different ways in which to provide this information.

Examples

In the article "Contraceptive Dynamics in Guatemala," Jane Bertrand, Eric Seiber, and Gabriela Escudero (2001) discuss various determinants that affect the use of contraceptives between two main ethnic groups in Guatemala: Mayan (indigenous) and Ladinos (a mixture of Spanish and Mayan).

In "Caring for Cambodian Refugees in the Emergency Department," Julie Miller (1995) presents some common Cambodian cultural beliefs about health care.

In the article "Fright Illness in Hmong Children" by Lisa Capps (1999), the author discusses the health problem known as fright illness that children in the Hmong community experience.

The author Judy Mill (2001) of the article "I'm Not a 'Basabasa' Woman: An Explanatory Model of HIV Illness in Ghanaian Women" explores Ghanaians' beliefs about HIV illness and the problems that HIV patients encounter.

The main idea of Mary Ann Hautman (1996) in "Changing Womanhood: Perimenopause among Filipina-Americans" is to understand the experiences of Filipina-Americans dealing with perimenopause.

Including the Title of the Journal

The introductory sentence can also include the title of the journal the article was published in, as in these examples:

Examples

The article "Illness and Treatment Perceptions of Ethiopian Immigrants and Their Doctors in Israel" by Marian Reiff and Havan Zakut, published in the *American Journal of Public Health* in 1999, discusses a research study that analyzes problems of understanding between immigrant patients and doctors.

The article "Somali Refugee Women's Experiences of Maternity Care in West London: A Case Study," written by Kate Bulman and Christine McCourt and published in *Critical Public Health* in 2002, is about a case study that was done with 12 Somali women and their experiences with maternity services while living in London.

As always, you need to make sure that the grammar of the resulting sentence is correct. One way is to temporarily remove all of the phrases and clauses inside commas. In other words, look at the **main clause** first and make sure it is a complete sentence. Then, add the rest of the information back into the sentence. For example, the main clause in the above example is:

The article . . . is about a case study that was done with 12 Somali women and their experiences with maternity services while living in London.

The rest of the sentence, besides the title of the article, has been added to the sentence as a **dependent clause.** The dependent clause is separated from the main clause by commas:

, written by Kate Bulman and Christine McCourt and published in *Critical Public Health* in 2002

Choosing Verbs

When you introduce your source or refer to the author in the summary itself, choose carefully the verbs you use. Your choice of verb will depend on the author's intention and on your purpose in referring to the idea. Some of the most frequently used verbs are listed.

When an author has a *neutral stance* toward the ideas expressed in his or her writing, you could refer to those ideas using these verbs:

ask	*explore*	*note*
describe	*find*	*observe*
discuss	*focus*	*point out*
emphasize	*identify*	*say*
establish	*illustrate*	*show*
examine	*indicate*	*write*
explain		

Some verbs are more appropriate for expressing an author's point of view or stance toward an idea. If the author is *claiming or asserting something to be true* or is trying to *convince you of the truth of his or her ideas,* you could use these verbs:

argue	*contend*	*propose*
assert	*declare*	*state*
assume	*insist*	*stress*
claim	*maintain*	*suggest*
conclude	*proclaim*	

If the author *states his or her opinion,* you could introduce their ideas with these verbs:

acknowledge	*advise*	*doubt*
admit	*believe*	*endorse*
advocate	*caution*	*recommend*
affirm	*condone*	*think*

Activity

In each example, circle the verb that is used to refer to the author's ideas. Analyze the choice of verb. Does it suggest the author has a neutral stance toward his or her ideas? Or is the author making an assertion of truth? Or is the author stating an opinion?

1. In the article "Fright Illness in Hmong Children" by Lisa Capps (1999), the author believes that children in the Hmong community experience health problems due to fright illness.
2. In "Changing Womanhood: Perimenopause among Filipina-Americans," Mary Ann Hautman (1996) describes what Filipina-Americans in perimenopause generally experience.
3. Calvillo and Flaskerud (1991) claim that many Hispanics believe "one's fate is to suffer in this world."
4. The author Judy Mill (2001) of the article "I'm Not a 'Basabasa' Woman: An Explanatory Model of HIV Illness in Ghanaian Women" explores what Ghanaians believe about HIV illness and the problems that HIV patients encounter.

Consider the effect these verbs have on the tone of the summary. What effect would a different kind of verb have? Substitute another kind of verb in each of these examples and discuss the different effects.

Writing a Summary and Critique

Your first writing assignment in this unit is to write a summary and critique of a nursing research article. A **summary** is a condensed version of an article. It includes paraphrasing of points from the original article. It can also include a few quotes of text that cannot be effectively paraphrased. Since a summary is supposed to be much shorter than the original article, it does not begin with a separate paragraph for the introduction, but rather with just an introductory statement. Likewise, it does not end with a separate paragraph for the conclusion, but with just a concluding statement. A **critique** is an evaluation of the article for its strengths and weaknesses.

Summarizing an article allows you to demonstrate your understanding of its content; critiquing the article allows you to demonstrate your ability to think critically about its content.

Guidelines for Writing a Summary

Follow these guidelines in writing a summary.

1. **Include only the main ideas of the article.** Key details may be included if they are particularly illustrative of main points. Paraphrase the main ideas; in other words, put them into your own words. Remember that you need to change the structure and wording of the entire sentence, not just a word or two to avoid plagiarizing. If you choose to quote from the article, quote selectively and sparingly.

2. **Use transitions to show the relationships between the main ideas in your summary.**

3. **In the first sentence of your summary, include the complete title of article, first and last names of author(s), name of journal where the article was published, date of publication of the journal, and topic of the article.** Make sure your introductory statement is grammatically complete and accurate.

4. **Refer occasionally to the author, using the last name only.** Vary the verbs that you use.

5. **Provide a concluding statement that summarizes the main point of the article.**

Requirements for documentation in a summary are different than for a research paper, which draws material from multiple outside sources. Since the only outside source for a summary is the original article, **you do not need to provide citations for paraphrased material** in the summary. However, you need to provide bibliographic information about the article at the very beginning of your summary in an introductory statement, and refer to the author(s) periodically throughout the summary. For quoted material, you do need to provide citations, but the citations should include only the page number in parentheses, not the author's last name and date of publication.

Provide complete bibliographic information for the article in a reference list at the end of the paper, in APA format.

A good test of your summary is to give it to someone who has not read the original article. Ask the person to read your summary and tell you what he or she understood from it. Is his or her understanding of the article consistent with yours? If not, discuss your different interpretations to pinpoint weaknesses in your summary.

Developing Your Critique

Some of your critique can reinforce or build on points that were made in the discussion section of the article, in particular the implications (for strengths of the study) and limitations (for weaknesses of the study). Recommendations for future research that would address limitations of the study could also be included.

In addition, questions that you could consider in developing your critique for the assignment on page 100 include:

- Did the article accurately reflect the beliefs and/or practices of your cultural group, or did it stereotype?
- Did the study accomplish what it was intended to? If not, were there flaws in the design of the study or the procedure used?
- Were the results of the study appropriately interpreted? If not, what alternate explanations would you suggest?

Maintaining an Objective Voice

Even though a critique represents your own ideas about the article, you should maintain an objective voice, that is, you should not use the personal pronoun *I,* as in *I think,* or possessive adjectives, such as: *in my opinion.* In nursing courses, *I* is acceptable only in personal, reflective writing.

In the example, the writer has made it clear what she agrees or disagrees with, but without using personal pronouns or possessive adjectives. Words that convey agreement or disagreement or that are evaluative in some way are italicized.

Example

The results of the study done by Liamputtong (2003) are *very compelling.* Overall, there were some *strengths and weaknesses* in the study. Some of the *strengths* were. . . . Even though there were *strengths,* there were also some *weaknesses* in the study.

Activity

In these excerpts, circle the words that convey the author's agreement or disagreement or that are evaluative in some way.

1. Even though the surveys used in the study (Bertrand, Seiber, & Escudero, 2001) were reliable and included large sample groups, it is questionable whether or not the participants represented the entire population. One of the weaknesses of the survey is that when the authors classified Guatemalans into two groups, they did not include a third group: the Burgesses.

2. Overall, Miller (1995) points out common Cambodian health care values and beliefs. Information regarding wind illness along with self-care techniques are described accurately. As a registered nurse, Miller provides excellent suggestions on how to be an effective caregiver for Cambodian patients. However, Miller misinterprets the use of the coining and cupping techniques. For instance, cupping is only used to treat headaches. Also, cooking oil and wax are rarely used as a lubricant during coining. In addition, Miller's findings were not based upon cultural research of the Cambodian ethnic groups. The author failed to provide statistics from past research findings. Her conclusions seem to be based only upon her experiences as a registered nurse.

Writing in Nursing: Summarizing and Critiquing Research

Summarize and critique an article from a nursing journal about your native cultural group and their experiences with health care in the United States or elsewhere, following the guidelines provided on pages 100–101. The article you select for this assignment should be handed in with your summary and critique.

Locating an Appropriate Article

First, find an article on the topic. If your native culture is well represented in the United States or in another country of migration (e.g., Canada, United Kingdom, Australia, Israel, etc.), you will most likely find several interesting articles to choose from. However, if you are unable to locate such an article, look for articles about your cultural group and some aspect of their health care in your native country.

It may also be that if you are from a smaller cultural group, you will need to locate articles using a broader cultural label or different country of migration. For example, if you are from Ecuador and are unable to find any articles about the health care experiences of Ecuadorians in North America, you may need to look for articles about health care experiences of South Americans or Latinos in the United States. Or, if you are from Kenya and are unable to find articles about the health care experiences of Kenyans in the United States, you may need to look for articles about the health care experiences of Kenyans in the United Kingdom or in Kenya itself.

The article must report on primary research or an actual research study that the authors of the article conducted; it cannot just discuss research studies that others have done. The methodology used in the research study can be either quantitative or qualitative. Quantitative methodology uses numbers to understand ideas, whereas in qualitative research, broad conceptual categories are explored through interviews, observations, and document analysis. (See pages 161 and 180 in Unit 5 for a discussion of quantitative and qualitative research methodology.) Articles based on qualitative research may be easier to read and understand, as qualitative research does not involve statistical analysis. However, it may be more difficult to summarize an article based on qualitative research, as the discussion of findings is usually longer and more detailed.

The article should be fairly recent, preferably published within the past five years, but certainly within the past ten years. Research studies that are more than five years old may be considered out of date, especially if there have been more recent studies done since. The exception is studies on cultural beliefs and practices in health care, for which the ten-year rule usually applies.

Locate articles in CINAHL that you could use for this assignment. List all keywords or combinations of keywords that you tried? ________________

____

Which ones were the most productive? ________________

____

How many hits were on your longest list? ________________

____

Explain your Search History and show a copy of your Search Results to your instructor.

Once you have conducted your search and have a list of articles, read through the abstracts of the articles that sound the most interesting. Ask these questions to determine which articles meet the criteria for the assignment and to decide which one to choose for this assignment.

1. Does the article address a health care issue in an immigrant community in the United States or elsewhere?
2. Is the article based on primary research?
3. Is the nature of the study interesting to you and not too difficult to understand?
4. Is the article from a nursing journal?

Reading and Understanding Research

Reading research articles is an important but challenging skill in nursing. It often takes several readings to understand a research-based article thoroughly. Apply the reading and study strategies discussed in Unit 1 (see pages 2–16) to help you understand the main points of the article you have selected for this assignment.

On a separate sheet of paper, outline the research study, using this template. This outline is designed for a quantitative research study, but it could be adapted for use with a qualitative study.

Outline of Quantitative Research Study

I. Purpose of the Study
II. Methodology
  A. Participants
  B. Instrument
  C. Procedure
III. Data Analysis
IV. Results of the Study
V. Discussion
  A. Conclusion
  B. Implications
  C. Limitations of the Study
  D. Recommendations

Developing Your Writing Skills

To develop your writing skills, you need to trust in the process of writing. You must also learn to recognize the needs of your reader.

The first step in becoming a more effective writer is to think of writing as a process that involves revising your writing multiple times.

When you begin to write a paper, you may not always know what you're going to say or where you're going to end. Even if you have very specific guidelines for what should be included in a paper, you may not know how you're going to satisfy each of those requirements. But, when you begin to write, your brain will start to generate ideas. Those ideas will lead to other ideas, usually better ideas than the ones you began with, like peeling off the outer leaves of lettuce that are sometimes wilted or crinkled around the edges, so you can get to the newer, tastier leaves inside.

Writing, then, is not just a way of communicating or documenting information; it is also a tool for thinking and learning. Each revision of a paper will improve not only the quality of your writing, but more importantly the quality of your thinking, which is at the heart of good writing.

Skilled writers anticipate the questions and concerns their readers are likely to have and address them during the revision process.

This ability of writers to anticipate the needs of readers is not automatic; it must be developed. Novice writers must learn how to distance themselves from their writing and see it through the eyes of potential readers. To help develop this skill, you will meet with classmates in small groups to review the rough drafts of your papers and to give each other feedback. Your instructor may also give you feedback at this or a subsequent stage of writing.

As you revise your rough drafts based on the feedback you have been given, you will begin to see what others have not understood and begin to anticipate the needs of your readers. When you give feedback to your peers, you will be helping them to develop this same awareness and skill. Eventually, with enough practice, you will be able to distance yourself from your own writing to evaluate its effectiveness.

Talking about a topic helps to understand it and write about it more effectively. The peer review process and oral presentations/discussion activities are two ways in which spoken fluency can help develop proficiency in written, academic English.

When you meet in small groups to review each other's rough drafts, talking about your paper helps you better understand what it is you're trying to communicate on paper. It also helps you find the language you need to put your thoughts down more easily and accurately on paper.

Writing about a topic is much easier after you have had a chance to talk about it with others or to present it orally to others. Discussion activities help you build on your spoken fluency to develop your proficiency in written, academic English.

Pre-Writing Activities: Discussion Questions

Before you begin reading and writing about culture and nursing, discuss in small groups what you already know about this topic. Form groups with classmates who do not have the same cultural background.

1. What is culture? Write a definition. What are the different components of culture? Make a list.
2. How does culture affect nursing? Provide specific examples from what you have heard or experienced.
3. To what extent does nursing currently tolerate, encourage, and/or incorporate culturally diverse perspectives and approaches to health and illness? Provide specific examples from what you have heard or experienced.
4. Have you or members of your family or cultural community experienced conflict with the U.S. health care system? If so, describe an experience. What was the belief, value, or practice that came into conflict between your native or home culture and the U.S. health care system?
5. How did this experience affect members of your family or community? Did such experiences influence your decision to become a nurse? If so, in what way?

Readings about Culture and Nursing

This chapter includes excerpts from two readings about culture and nursing. These readings will provide you with ideas and information to include in writing about culture and nursing.

Reading 3.1

Culture and Heritage*

Barbara Kozier, MN, RN; Glenora Erb, BSN, RN;
Audrey Berman, PhD, RN, AOCN; Shirlee J. Snyder, EdD, RN

Culture can be defined as the nonphysical traits—such as values, beliefs, attitudes, and customs—that are shared by a group of people and passed from one generation to the next (Spector, 2000). Culture also defines how health is perceived; how health care information is received; how rights and protections are exercised; what is considered to be a health problem, and how symptoms and concerns about the health problem are expressed; who should provide treatment and how; and what kind of treatment should be given.

Nurses must be aware that, although people from a given group share certain beliefs, values, and experiences, often there is also widespread **intragroup** diversity. Major differences within groups may be due to such factors as age, gender, level of education, socioeconomic status, and area of origin in the home country (rural or urban). Such factors influence the client's beliefs about health and illness, practices, help-seeking behaviors, and expectations of nurses. For these reasons, effort must be made and care taken to avoid the stereotyping of people from a specific group.

National Standards for Culturally and Linguistically Appropriate Services in Health Care

The composition of the population of the United States has changed over the past 30 years. Given the ongoing changes in the population, *National Standards for Culturally and Linguistically Appropriate Services in Health Care* (CLAS) have been created (Office of Minority Health [OMH], 2001). Culture and language have a considerable impact on how clients access and respond to health care services. Furthermore, to ensure equal access to quality health care by diverse populations, health care organizations and nurses should "promote and support, the attitudes, behaviors, knowledge, and skills necessary for staff to work respectfully and effectively with clients and each other in a culturally diverse work environment" (OMH, 2001, p. 7). The standards are based on key laws, regulations, contracts, and standards currently in use by federal and state agencies and other national organizations to evaluate the cultural quality of care.

Culturally Competent Nursing Care

Culturally competent nursing is critical to meeting the complex nursing care needs of a given person, family, and community. It is the provision of nursing care across cultural boundaries and takes into account the context in which the client lives as well as the situations in which the client's health problems arise. It goes much further than both culturally sensitive and culturally appropriate care (see definitions below), as it requires an understanding and integration of the *total context* of the client, as well as knowledge, attitudes, and skills in the delivery of care.

*From Kozier, Barbara; Erb, Glenora; Berman, Audrey J.; Snyder, Shirlee, FUNDAMENTALS OF NURSING: CONCEPTS, PROCEDURES, & PRACTICES, 7th Edition, © 2004. Reprinted by permission of Pearson Education, Inc., Upper Saddle River, NJ.

- **Culturally sensitive** implies that the nurse possesses some basic *knowledge* of and constructive *attitudes* toward the health traditions observed among the diverse cultural groups found in the setting in which they are practicing.
- **Culturally appropriate** implies that the nurse applies the underlying background *knowledge* that must be possessed to provide a given client with the best possible health care.
- **Culturally competent** implies that within the delivered care the nurse understands and attends to the *total context* of the client's situation and uses a complex combination of *knowledge, attitudes*, and *skills*.

In order to meet the mandates of the CLAS standards, nursing practice must become culturally competent. Conflicts in the health care delivery arenas are often the result of cultural misunderstandings. Culturally competent care enables the nurse to understand, from a cultural perspective, the manifestations of the client's health beliefs and practices.

Health Beliefs and Practices

Andrews and Boyle (2002) describe three views of health beliefs: magico-religious, scientific, and holistic. In the **magico-religious health belief** view, health and illness are controlled by supernatural forces. The client may believe that illness is the result of "being bad" or opposing God's will. Getting well is also viewed as dependent on God's will. The client may make statements such as, "If it is God's will, I will recover" or "What did I do wrong to be punished with cancer?" Some cultures believe that magic can cause illness. A sorcerer or witch may put a spell or hex on the client. Some people view illness as possession by an evil spirit. Although these beliefs are not supported by **empirical evidence,** clients who believe that such things can cause illness may in fact become ill as a result. Such illnesses may require magical treatments in addition to scientific treatments. For example, a man who experiences gastric distress, headaches, and hypertension after being told that a spell has been placed on him may recover only if the spell is removed by the culture's healer.

The **scientific or biomedical health belief** is based on the belief that life and life processes are controlled by physical and biochemical processes that can be manipulated by humans (Andrews & Boyle, 2002). The client with this view will believe that illness is caused by germs, viruses, bacteria, or a breakdown of the human machine, the body. This client will expect a pill, or treatment, or surgery to cure health problems.

The **holistic health belief** holds that the forces of nature must be maintained in balance or harmony. Human life is one aspect of nature that must be in harmony with the rest of nature. When the natural balance or **harmony** is disturbed, illness results. The medicine wheel is an ancient symbol used by Native Americans of North and South America to express many concepts. For health and wellness, the medicine wheel teaches the four aspects of the individual's nature: the physical, the mental, the emotional, and the spiritual. The four dimensions must be in balance to be healthy. The medicine wheel can also be used to express the individual's relationship with the environment as a dimension of wellness.

The concept of **yin and yang** in the Chinese culture and the hot–cold theory of illness in many Spanish cultures are examples of holistic health beliefs. When a Chinese client has a yin illness or a "cold" illness, the treatment may include a yang or "hot" food (e.g., hot tea). For example, a Chinese client who has been diagnosed with cancer, a yin disease, will want to eat cultural foods that have yang properties.

What is considered hot or cold varies considerably across cultures. In many cultures, the mother who has just delivered a baby should be offered warm or hot foods and kept warm with blankets because childbirth is seen as a "cold" condition. Conventional scientific thought recommends cooling the body to reduce a fever. The physician may order liquids for the client and cool compresses to be applied to the forehead, the **axillae,** or the **groin.** Galanti (1997) states that many cultures believe that the best way to treat a fever is to "sweat it out." Clients from these cultures may want to cover up with several blankets, take hot baths, and drink hot beverages. The nurse must keep in mind that a treatment strategy that is consistent with the client's beliefs may have a better chance of being successful. For example, the Latino client who avoids "hot" foods when experiencing a stomach disturbance may be eating foods consistent with the bland diet that is normally prescribed by physicians.

Socio-cultural forces, such as politics, economics, geography, religion, and the predominant health care system, influence the client's health status and health care behavior. For example, people who have limited access to scientific health care may turn to folk medicine or folk healing. **Folk medicine** is defined as those beliefs and practices relating to illness prevention and healing that derive from cultural traditions rather than from modem medicine's scientific base. Many students can recall special teas or "cures" used by older family members to prevent or treat colds, fevers, indigestion, and other common health problems. People also continue to use chicken soup as a treatment for influenza (the "flu").

Why do individuals use these non-traditional folk healing methods? Folk medicine, in contrast to biomedical health care, is thought to be more **humanistic.** The **consultation** and treatment takes place in the community of the recipient, frequently in the home of the healer. It is less expensive than scientific or biomedical care because the health problem is identified primarily through conversation with the client and the family. The healer often prepares the treatments, for example, teas to be **ingested, poultices** to be applied, or **charms** or **amulets** to be worn. A frequent component of treatment is some ritual practice on the part of the healer or the client to cause healing to occur. Because folk healing is more culturally based, it is often more comfortable and less frightening for the client.

It is important for the nurse to obtain information about folk or family healing practices that may have been used before the client decided to seek Western medical treatment. Often clients are reluctant to share **home remedies** with health care professionals for fear of being laughed at or rebuked.

Family Patterns

The family is the basic unit of society. Cultural values can determine communication within the family group, the norm for family size, and the roles of specific family members. In some families, the man is considered the provider and decision maker. The woman may need to consult her husband before making decisions about her medical treatment or the treatment of her children. Some families are **matriarchal;** that is, the mother or grandmother is viewed as the leader of the family and is usually the decision maker. The nurse needs to identify who has the "authority" to make decisions in a client's family. If the decision maker is someone other than the client, the nurse needs to include that person in health care discussions.

The value placed on children and elders within a society is culturally derived. In some cultures, children are not disciplined, by spanking or other forms of physical punishment. Rather, children are allowed to interact with their environment while caregivers provide subtle direction to prevent harm or injury. In other cultures, elderly people are considered the holders of the culture's wisdom and are therefore highly respected. Responsibility for caring for older relatives is determined by cultural practices. In many cultures, older relatives who cannot live independently often live with a married son or daughter and family.

Cultural gender-role behavior may also affect nurse-client interactions. In some countries, men dominate and women have little status. Men from these countries may not accept instruction from a female nurse or physician but will be receptive to the same instruction given by a male physician or nurse. Some cultures have a prevailing concept of **machismo,** or male superiority. The positive aspects of machismo require that the adult man provide for and protect his family, including extended family members. The woman is expected to maintain the home and raise the children.

Cultural family values may also dictate the extent of the family's involvement in the hospitalized client's care. In some cultures, the nuclear and the extended family will want to visit for long periods and participate in care. In other cultures, the entire **clan** may want to visit and participate in the client's care. This can cause concern on nursing units with strict visiting policies. The nurse should evaluate the positive benefits of family participation in the client's care and modify visiting policies as appropriate.

Cultures that value the needs of the extended family as much as those of the individual may hold the belief that personal and family information must stay within the family. Some cultural groups are very reluctant to disclose family information to outsiders, including health care professionals. This attitude can present difficulties for health care professionals who require knowledge of family interaction patterns to help clients with emotional problems.

References

Andrews, M. M., & Boyle, J. S. (2002). *Transcultural concepts in nursing care* (4th ed.). Philadelphia: Lippincott Williams & Wilkins.

Galanti, G. (1997). *Caring for patients from different cultures: Case studies from American hospitals* (2nd ed.). Philadelphia: University of Pennsylvania Press.

Office of Minority Health. (2001). *National standards for culturally and linguistically appropriate services in health care.* Washington, DC: U.S. Department of Health and Human Services.

Spector, R. E. (2000). *Cultural diversity in health and illness* (5th ed.). Upper Saddle River, NJ: Prentice Hall.

Activity: Vocabulary Development

Reading 3.1 contains many socio-cultural terms that are used to explain health beliefs and practices. Add the words you do not know to your dictionary, following the guidelines on page 33. Use a college-level English dictionary to look up the words you do not know. Use 10–15 new words in answering the discussion questions.

Comprehension and Discussion Questions

The questions ask you to relate ideas from the reading to your own personal experiences and cultural context, as an individual and as a member of a family and community.

1. What are some ways in which there is intra-group variation within cultural communities? Can you think of ways in which you and members of your family and/or cultural community are different from one another? Provide specific examples. Why do you think there are these differences?

2. Access online the *National Standards for Culturally and Linguistically Appropriate Services in Health Care* (CLAS). How many standards are there? Which do you think are the most important? To what extent have you and your family received culturally and linguistically appropriate health care services in the United States or elsewhere? Provide specific examples.

3. Of the three health beliefs described by Andrews and Boyle (2002)—the magico-religious, scientific/biomedical, and holistic—which view do you believe in? Your family? Your cultural community? Provide specific examples. Are your views the same as your family or cultural community? Why or why not?

4. Re-read the example on page 92. How would you explain to the nurse why Mrs. Chen gave her son, Phillip, cold tea?

5. Do you, your family, and/or cultural community practice folk medicine? Provide specific examples. Are your practices the same as your family or cultural community? Why or why not?

6. In your family, who makes the decisions with regard to health care? Does that conflict with how health care decisions are usually made in the United States? If so, in what ways? Provide specific examples.

7. When a member of your family is in the hospital, who comes to visit? How long do they stay? Does your family or community's practices conflict with U.S. hospital visitation policies? If so, in what ways? Provide specific examples.

Reading 3.2

Review of Literature on Culture and Pain of Adults with Focus on Mexican-Americans

Evelyn Ruiz Calvillo, MSN, RN, Associate Professor, Department of Nursing, California State University, Los Angeles

Jacquelyn H. Flaskerud, PhD, RN, FAAN, Professor, School of Nursing, University of California, Los Angeles

Cultural groups in the United States are sometimes characterized according to their ability to tolerate pain. These characterizations often approach stereotypes in statements such as "Mexican Americans have a low pain tolerance" or "Italian Americans are very dramatic about their pain" or "Jewish Americans complain a lot about pain" or "Asian Americans do not express their pain." Because nurses are often in primary contact with patients, they may be the most likely of all health professionals to make assessments of patients' pain and to manage their pain. Nurses are in a position to make judgments about the **severity** of the patient's pain and whether or not the patient should receive pain medication. Often these judgments are influenced by ethnic stereotypes and the clock. That is, nurses make their decisions based on their own impressions of what a person's **pain threshold** ought to be (related to their own cultural values) and on when the patient received his or her last pain medication. It is important, therefore, that nurses understand both the phenomenon of pain and the role that culture plays in the perception and expression of pain. This understanding is necessary to the nurse's accurate and appropriate assessment and management of patients' pain.

The purposes of this paper are to review the general research literature on culture and pain in adults in the United States; specific studies of Mexican-American responses to pain; and studies of nurses' evaluation of patients' pain. Implications are drawn for transcultural nursing practice and suggestions are made for future transcultural nursing research among Mexican-Americans based on the studies reviewed.

Conceptual Framework: Culture and Pain

The role that culture plays in the perception of pain both by people from different cultures and nurses may be conceptualized by integrating concepts of transcultural nursing (Leininger, 1976, 1977, 1979, 1984), traditional beliefs about health and illness of a specific ethnocultural group, and the gate control theory of pain (Melzack, 1983). Transcultural nursing draws from the framework of the relationship between culture and pain. Leininger states that culture is the "blueprint for thought and action" (1976, p. 9) and is a dominant force in determining health and illness behaviors.

Traditional beliefs provide culture-specific examples of values, attitudes and experiences. **Indigenous** or traditional beliefs affect the perception of health and illness which often includes expected behaviors in response to illness and pain. Beliefs are important constructs which lie at the core of "culture" and which are seen as antecedents of behavior (Castro et al., 1984).

For example, in many Hispanic cultures the value of suffering and the concept of **fatalism** are accepted beliefs with religious **undertones.** Many Hispanic persons believe that life has many difficulties which must be accepted without complaints. One's **fate** is to suffer in this world and "submit with patience to one's **allotted** measure of suffering" (Calatrello, 1980). If a person is ill, that person bears the illness with dignity and courage. Many are able to progress through an illness or through a recovery period with this attitude because "everything is in the hands of God" (Calatrello, 1980).

The gate control theory of pain proposed by Melzack and Wall (Melzack, 1983) provides an explanation of the relationship between pain and culture. These investigators established that pain is not just a **physiological** response to tissue damage, but that psychological variables such as behavioral and emotional responses expected and accepted by one's cultural group influence the perception of pain. These expectations are stored in the brain and in cultural experiences and are capable of influencing the **transmission** of painful stimuli throughout the individual's life.

Gate control theory suggests that transmission of pain impulses can be **modulated** or altered by a **gating mechanism** composed of **blocking cells** all along the **nervous system.** When these cells are **activated,** the gate is closed and pain impulses do not flow to the brain. If these cells are not stimulated, impulses get through the open gate to the brain. Similar **pain-inhibiting** mechanisms exist in descending **nerve fibers** in the **thalamus** and the **cerebral cortex.** These areas of the brain regulate processes related to thoughts, emotions, and past experiences. These structures send messages to open or close the gate. When pain is occurring, the individual's thoughts, cultural beliefs and values, and memories can influence whether pain impulses reach the level of awareness (Meinhart & McCaffery, 1983).

Although pain is held to be basically a physiological phenomenon, the meaning and responses to pain may be determined by cultural experiences and beliefs. Culture is an important variable in determining an individual's behavioral response to pain. Leininger (1979) states that a person's reaction to illness, health maintenance, bodily discomforts, and caring and curing practices are linked with cultural beliefs, values, and experiences. A person learns what is expected and accepted by his or her culture; this learning includes reactions to painful experiences. Perception, expression, and management of pain are all **embedded** in a cultural context. The definition of pain, just like that of health and illness, is culturally determined (Ludwig-Beymer, 1989). According to Meinhart and McCaffery (1983) cultural expectations may specify: (a) different reactions according to age, sex, and occupation, (b) what treatment to seek, (c) the **intensity** and **duration** of pain that should be tolerated, (d) what responses should be made, (e) who to report to when pain occurs, and (f) what types of pain require attention. It is possible that a patient's cultural background influences not only attitudes towards pain but the **overt** response to it as well.

Transcultural Pain Studies

In the United States, the cultural beliefs of Anglo-Americans are considered **dominant** in spite of the fact that there is little social research done on them (Harwood, 1981). This group is selected as the reference group in transcultural comparison studies because their social and cultural behaviors represent the accepted pattern (Castro et al., 1984; Winsberg & Greenlick, 1967; Zborowski, 1952, 1969). Zborowski (1952) conducted a classic and the best known study of pain in European-origin ethnic groups. The study described the dominant culture values of pain experience which are still used today. The Anglo-American patient reports pain and is able to give a detailed description of it; however, the person usually demonstrates few emotional side reactions to pain. When in pain, the Anglo-American tries to remain calm, avoiding complaining, crying, screaming, or other **manifestations** of pain.

Meinhart and McCaffery (1983) reported that among Anglo-Americans **vocalizations** are viewed as useless but an occasional jerk or "ouch" are considered acceptable. When the patient is in severe pain, an attempt is made to withdraw in order to minimize pain and reduce pity. **Stoicism** is valued; there is pride in being the good patient, i.e., one who does not annoy anyone with his or her pain experience. The pain reaction of this group is the cultural model for the dominant society. Ideal patients are expected to behave and react to pain based on this model whether or not they are of Anglo-American origin.

Zborowski's early study, conducted in 1952, has been pertinent to subsequent cross-cultural studies on the influence of culture on pain. The study described the pain response patterns in Anglo-Americans, Italians, Jews, and Irish. Age, education, occupation, socioeconomic status, the disease causing the pain, and ethnicity were compared. Zborowski found differences in the pain response among the four groups and concluded that culture and social conditioning played an important role in pain behavior. He suggested that **patterned** attitudes toward pain exist in every culture. Appropriate and inappropriate expressions of pain are culturally **prescribed.** Cultural traditions dictate whether to expect and tolerate pain in certain situations and how to behave during a painful experience (Ludwig-Beymer, 1989).

Hospital staff in Zborowski study tended to support the Anglo-American response to pain and to characterize the other groups as overreacting, emotional, and complaining. Zborowski disagreed with this interpretation considering it too simplistic. He reached two conclusions based on his study: 1) similar reactions (behaviors, vocalizations) to pain demonstrated by members of different ethnocultural groups do not necessarily reflect similar attitudes toward pain; and 2) reactive patterns similar in their manifestations (e.g., crying, moaning or stoicism) may have different functions in various cultures (Zborowski, 1952).

Using Zborowski's hypotheses and the same four ethnic groups, Sternback and Tursky (1965) conducted **threshold, magnitude** estimation, and **physiological reactivity** studies of responses to electric shock. The groups were controlled on a number of physical and social variables (sex, age, height, weight, social class). They differed in religion and generation of immigration (although all subjects were U.S. born). The groups did not differ in **pain threshold** (ability to perceive and report the pain sensation); however, they differed significantly in **pain tolerance** (magnitude or severity of pain tolerated). Anglo-Americans had the highest pain tolerance mean scores followed by Jews, Irish, and Italians, in that order. The investigators concluded that there were attitudinal differences in pain sensitivity and tolerance.

Wolff and Langley (1979) reviewed all relevant studies on cultural factors and the response to pain up to that date. Results of the various studies they reviewed were **equivocal.** Often studies were difficult to compare because of 1) the different methods used to **induce** pain, 2) **laboratory** versus **field conditions,** and 3) lack of controls. For example, an early study which found differences in the pain response of Black and White Americans was **contradicted** by another study of these same groups when social class was **controlled.** A study by Flannery and colleagues (1981) supported the importance of controlling social class. They found no difference in response to **episiotomy** pain among Black, Italian, Jewish, Irish, and Anglo-Saxon Protestant patients when education was controlled. Although none of the studies allowed for a definitive conclusion about differences in pain sensation among ethnic groups, Wolff and Langley (1979) determined that attitudinal factors influence the pain response (the reaction to pain or expression of pain) of different cultures.

Pain Response in Mexican-Americans

Mexican-Americans are a diverse group and there are many intragroup differences among them that could affect responses to pain. There are a large number of today's Mexican-Americans who no longer believe or practice the folk medicine of their **forefathers** (Gonzalez-Swafford & Gutierrez, 1983). Still there is a large percentage of Mexican-Americans who hold traditional beliefs. More intense **adherence** to the Mexican culture seems to produce more traditional health behavior (Castro et al., 1984; Harwood, 1981).

The traditional beliefs of Mexican-Americans provide one part of a conceptual framework for understanding the relationship of culture and pain in this group. As noted earlier, Calatrello (1980) found that when an Hispanic individual is ill, the person bears the illness with dignity and courage; this is because many Hispanics believe that difficulties are part of life and must be accepted without complaints. Stoicism is valued, and many times signs and symptoms of pain are not acknowledged because lack of **stamina** is considered a sign of weakness.

Self-control is a practice common to the Mexican-American who is experiencing pain. Castro and colleagues (1984) found that the concept of self-control is an important element in the Mexican culture. Self-control *(controlarse)* includes: 1) the ability to withstand stress in times of **adversity** *(aguantarse);* 2) a passive **resignation** in which the person accepts his or her fate *(resignarse);* or 3) a more active cognitive **coping** which means working through a problem *(sobreponerse).*

Many Mexican-American patients, especially women, **moan** when uncomfortable. Consequently, they are often identified by the nursing staff as complainers who cannot tolerate pain (Orque et al., 1983). These investigators stated that in the Mexican culture, crying out with pain is an acceptable expression and not **synonymous** with an inability to tolerate pain. Crying out with pain does not necessarily indicate either that the pain experience is severe or that the person is experiencing a loss of self-control. Neither does it mean that the patient expects the nurse to intervene. Some patients may react to mild pain by crying or moaning and others may suppress overt behaviors with severe pain. Neither expression or behavior is a demand for nursing management of the pain without further nursing assessment of the situation. Zborowski's (1952, 1969) conclusions are especially relevant to this situation. He made the point that similar **patterns** do not necessarily have the same **function.** Nurses operating from the dominant culture model of response to pain might interpret the pattern of crying and moaning as an inability to tolerate pain and a request for **intervention.** In the Mexican culture, however, the pattern of crying and moaning might have the function for the patient of relieving pain rather than the function of communicating a request for intervention. This example points out clearly that any attempt to **delineate** cultural factors in the pain response should be made within the wider context of cultural attitudes and behaviors.

In cross-cultural studies regarding how patients viewed and described their pain (Kalish & Reynolds, 1976; Meinhart & McCaffery, 1983), descriptions by Hispanic subjects were consistent with the beliefs of fatalism, stoicism and self-restraint reported as valued in the Hispanic culture. In a study conducted by Lipton and Marbach (1980), Hispanics were less willing to admit loss of control and less likely to describe their pain as **unbearable** (Meinhart & McCaffery, 1983). Their descriptions were consistent with the beliefs of the Hispanic culture that stoicism and self-control are valued.

Among Anglo-Americans and especially Anglo American nurses, the stereotype exists that Mexican Americans cannot stand pain. Despite the lack of any evidence to support it, Perez-Stable (1987) notes that Mexican-American patients are often characterized as dramatic, emotional and complainers.

Evaluation of Pain Response by Nurses

Health caregivers' views of pain have been analyzed in many studies in which the culture of the patient and the nurse did not differ or in which culture was not considered as a variable. There have been consistent differences between patients and health care staff in assessing the severity of patients' pain (Teske et al., 1983), which generally resulted in more suffering for the patient (Cohen, 1980; Jacox, 1979; Teske et al., 1983). Regardless of culture, nurses gave less medication for pain than ordered and less medication than patients needed to **alleviate** their pain. Both nurses and physicians had a limited understanding of long-term **narcotic** use; they lacked knowledge of current pain management techniques; and they **overestimated** the potential for **addiction** to **prescription** narcotics (Rankin & Snider, 1984).

Streltzer and Wade (1981) studied **post-cholecystectomy** pain in Whites, Hawaiians, and Asians. They noted that nurses commonly limited the amount of **analgesic** administered to all their patients. However, some patients received fewer analgesics than others. This difference seemed to be based on ethnicity, with less **vocal** ethnic groups (Asians) receiving the least medication. Several investigators have given explanations for nurses' **underestimation** and undertreatment of their patient's pain (Jacox, 1979; Meinhart & McCaffery, 1983). With repeated **exposure** to patient pain and suffering, nurses gradually become less sensitive to patients' complaints of pain. In addition, nurses fear causing **respiratory depression** in their patients and addiction. They also lack knowledge of basic **pharmacology** or fail to apply their knowledge.

Nursing staff in the studies cited tended to uphold the dominant culture values which strongly encourage stoicism during pain experiences and to believe that patients exaggerate their pain experiences. Davitz and Davitz (1981) studied nurses' attitudes toward pain and found that the patient's ethnicity was related to how much physical and psychological distress the nurse believed the patient was experiencing. Nurses thought that Jewish and Spanish-speaking patients expressed the most distress with pain and Anglo-Saxon patients the least. The nurses' own cultural background also influenced how much distress they thought patients were experiencing with pain. Nurses of Northern European and United States backgrounds thought patients were experiencing less physical pain and psychological distress, whereas nurses of Eastern and Southern European or African backgrounds thought patients were experiencing more pain and psychological distress. This was true regardless of the nurses' years of experience, position, and area of practice. These investigators concluded that nurses' judgments about the pain and distress suffered by patients are influenced by their own beliefs about suffering. Cultural factors, social class, religion, education, and ethnic background all played a role in nurses' inferences of patients' pain. Regardless of cultural background, however, all studies reviewed here showed that nurses and other medical staff consistently underestimated pain when compared to their patients' reports of pain.

Implications for Transcultural Nursing Practice

These studies suggest a need among nurses for transcultural knowledge of pain assessment and management. In making an assessment of a Mexican-American and his or her potential response to pain, the cultural beliefs, values and practices of the client must be assessed with respect to illness, suffering and pain.

An assessment of actual responses to pain should include gathering data on what a particular behavior and/or vocalization might mean in response to pain. For example, does it mean the pain is merely perceived or recognized? Or does it mean the pain is **intolerable?** Secondly, an assessment of actual response to pain should include gathering data on the function of particular behaviors and vocalizations, for example, crying and moaning. Is the function of these behaviors and vocalizations to relieve the pain? Or is the function to **signal** the nurse that pain intervention is being requested? Or is it something else?

The management of the patient's pain should include an assessment of the type of intervention the person desires. Does the patient wish traditional interventions, expressions of nurturance and compassion, psychological support, physical interventions (**soothing,** having **brow wiped,** relaxation)? cultural support? medication? or a combination of these? Does the patient value self-control and can the nurse assist the patient in practicing self-control if this is desired? The role of the family or social support network in providing any of these interventions should be assessed as well and **accommodations** made for family, friends and clergy to provide interventions. These are a few of the most obvious implications for transcultural nursing practice based on the studies of Mexican-Americans reviewed in this paper.

References

Calatrello, R. L. (1980). The Hispanic concept of illness: An obstacle to effective health care management? *Behavioral Medicine, 7*(11), 23–28.

Castro, F. G., Furth, P., & Karlow, H. (1984). The health beliefs of Mexican, Mexican-American, and Anglo-American women. *Hispanic Journal of Behavioral Sciences, 6*(4), 365–368.

Cohen, F. L. (1980). Postsurgical pain relief: Patients' status and nurses' medication choices. *Pain, 9*(1), 265–274.

Davitz, J. R., & Davitz, L. J. (1981). Influences on patients' pain and psychological distress. New York: Springer-Verlag.

Flannery, R. B., Sos, J., & McGovern, P. (1981). Ethnicity as a factor in the expression of pain. *Psychosomatics, 22*(1), 34–39, 45, 49–50.

Gonzalez-Swafford, M. L., & Gutierrez, M. G. (1983). Ethnomedical beliefs and practices of Mexican-Americans. *Nurse Practitioner, 8*(10), 29–34.

Harwood, A. (1981). *Ethnicity and medical care.* Cambridge: Harvard University Press.

Jacox, A. K. (1979). Assessing pain. *American Journal of Nursing, 79*(5), 895–900.

Kalish, R. A., & Reynolds, D. K. (1976). *Death and ethnicity: A psycho-cultural study.* Los Angeles: Ethel Percy Andrus Gerontology Center/ University of Southern California.

Leininger, M. (1976). *Trans-cultural health care issues and conditions.* Philadelphia: F.A. Davis.

Leininger, M. (1977). Cultural diversities of health and nursing care. *Nursing Clinics of North America, 12*(1), 5–18.

Leininger, M. (1979). *Trans-cultural nursing.* New York: Masson.

Leininger, M. (1984). Trans-cultural nursing: An overview. *Nursing Outlook, 32*(2), 72–73.

Lipton, J. A., & Marbach, J. J. (1980). Pain differences, similarities found. *Science News, 118,* 182–183.

Ludwig-Beymer, P. (1989). Trans-cultural aspects of pain. In J. S. Boyle & M. M. Andrews (Eds.), *Transcultural concepts in nursing care.* Glenview, IL: Scott-Foresman.

Meinhart, N. T., & McCaffery, M. (1983). *Pain: A nursing approach to assessment and analysis.* Norwalk, CT: Appleton-CenturyCrofts.

Melzack, R. (1983). *Pain measurement and assessment.* New York: Raven Press.

Orque, M., Bloch, B., & Monrroy, L. S. (1983). *Ethnic nursing care: A multicultural approach.* St. Louis: Mosby.

Perez-Stable, E. J. (1987). Issues in Latino healthcare. *Western Journal of Medicine, 139,* 820–828.

Rankin, M. A., & Snider, B. (1984). Nurses' perception of cancer patients' pain. *Cancer Nursing, 7*(2), 149–155.

Sternbach, R. A., & Tursky, B. (1965). Ethnic differences among housewives in psychophysical and skin potential response to electric shock. *Psychophysiology, 1,* 241–246.

Streltzer, J., & Wade, T. C. (1981). The influence of cultural group on the undertreatment of postoperative pain. *Psycho-somatic Medicine, 43*(5), 397–403.

Teske, K., Daut, R. L., & Cleeland, C. S. (1983). Relationships between nurses' observations and patients' self-reports of pain. *Pain, 16*(3), 286–296.

Winsberg, B., & Greenlick, M. (1967). Pain response in Negro and White obstetrical patients. *Journal of Health Social Behavior, 8,* 222–227.

Wolff, B. B., & Langley, S. (1979). Cultural factors and the response to pain. In D. Landy (Ed.), *Culture, disease, and healing* (pp. 313–319). New York: McMillan.

Zborowksi, M. (1952). Cultural components in responses to pain. *Journal of Social Issues, 8,* 16–30.

Zborowksi, M. (1969). *People in pain.* San Francisco: JosseyBass.

Activity: Vocabulary Development

Reading 3.2 contains many socio-cultural terms related to pain, words used to describe research, and specialized medical/nursing terms. Add the words to your dictionary that you do not know, following the guidelines on page 33. Use a medical English dictionary to look up medical/nursing terms and a college-level English dictionary to look up the research terms that you do not know. Use 10–15 new words in answering the discussion questions.

Comprehension and Discussion Questions

These questions ask you to locate important information in the article, as well as analyze carefully and think critically about information in the reading. In small groups, discuss your answers to these questions.

1. On page 112, the authors state: "Beliefs . . . lie at the core of 'culture' and . . . are seen as antecedents of behavior." Explain what this statement means. What are the beliefs about life, suffering, and fatalism in Hispanic cultures that are the "antecedents of behavior" regarding the response to pain in these cultures?
2. What is the gate control theory of pain? Why is it relevant in a discussion of culture and pain?
3. According to Zborowski's (1952) study, what is the Anglo-American response to pain? Why do you think the pain reaction of this group has been the cultural model or norm for all groups in the United States? Do you think the Anglo-American response to pain is still the cultural norm today? Why or why not?
4. The authors refer to the findings of one study that was "contradicted by another study of these same groups when *social class* was controlled" (page 114). They also refer to another study that found "no difference in response to episiotomy pain among Black, Italian, Jewish, Irish, and Anglo-Saxon Protestant patients when *education* was controlled" (page 114). Explain what it means when social class and education are controlled. Why are these findings significant in a discussion of culture and response to pain?
5. In the discussion of traditional health beliefs of Hispanics, why is it important to be stoic in Hispanic cultures? How is the stoicism of Hispanics different from the stoicism of Anglo-Americans in their response to pain?

6. On page 115, the authors state: "Many Mexican-American patients, especially women, moan when uncomfortable. . . . crying out with pain is [also] an acceptable expression." What do these behaviors usually mean within the context of Mexican-American culture? How are these behaviors frequently interpreted by nurses operating from the dominant cultural model?
7. Studies on pain response in Mexican Americans do not support the stereotype that "Mexican-Americans cannot stand pain" (page 115). In your opinion, why does the stereotype of Mexican-American patients as "dramatic, emotional and complainers" (page 115) exist despite the lack of evidence to support it?
8. How is pain responded to in your culture? What are the beliefs and attitudes toward pain in your culture that are the "antecedents of behavior"? Do these beliefs, attitudes, and behaviors toward pain vary among groups within your culture? In what ways? Are these beliefs, attitudes, and behaviors in the process of changing? Why or why not?
9. Studies have consistently found that regardless of culture, "nurses gave less medication for pain than ordered and less medication than patients needed to alleviate their pain" (page 115). What are the reasons given for these findings? Why are these findings significant?
10. What are the implications of the studies reviewed in this article (e.g., Streltzer & Wade, 1981; Davitz & Davitz, 1981) regarding how nurses should assess and manage a patient's response to pain?

Research-Based Writing Assignment

For your second writing assignment in this unit, write a five- to six-page research paper on cultural influences on nursing practice, using ideas and information from four or five written outside sources. For this assignment, apply the research skills and the research-based writing skills you have worked on in this unit.

For this paper, you will need to do some reading in the area of cultural diversity in nursing, also referred to as transcultural nursing. Follow the guidelines regarding the content and organization of the paper.

In the introduction:

- Define culture, using a definition from a nursing textbook.
- Explain the importance of cultural competence in nursing.
- State the purpose of the paper, which is to discuss cultural inferences on nursing practice; this is your **thesis statement**.

In the body:

- Discuss thoroughly three ways in which culture influences nursing, providing specific examples to support your points.
- Reflect on your own cultural background and how it may (or may not) influence you (positively and/or negatively) as a nurse in the United States or as a nurse who has been U.S. trained in your home country. Provide specific examples to support your points. Provide smooth, effective transitions from the introduction to the body of your paper and from the first part of your discussion to the second part, that is, from your discussion of how culture influences nursing, to how your cultural background may or may not influence you as a nurse.

In the conclusion:

- Provide clear connections between your reflection on how your cultural background may or may not influence you as a nurse and your discussion of how culture influences nursing. In other words, tie the second part of your paper back to the first part.

In-text citations and reference list:

- Use a writer's handbook or the *APA Publication Manual* to help you with the correct formatting for in-text citations and the reference list.

Before you turn in the final revision of your paper, review the checklist to evaluate your final draft. After the instructor has evaluated your paper, compare your evaluation of your paper with your instructor's. How similar were they? In what ways did they differ?

Journal Writing

Throughout the rest of the textbook, you are asked to reflect on culturally sensitive topics in nursing, such as mental illness and sexuality. Other assignments ask you to think critically about ethical dilemmas that may arise in nursing when providing care for clients whose beliefs, values, and practices concerning health issues conflict with those of the U.S. health care system. These journal assignments allow you to reflect on the cultural content of nursing, in particular your own cultural beliefs and values, and how they may or may not be consistent with the underlying beliefs, values, and practices in the U.S. health care system. These assignments also allow you to reflect on any difficulties you may anticipate as a future U.S. health care provider or elsewhere because of these differences.

For these assignments, you do not need to be concerned with the rules and conventions of academic writing, as discussed throughout this chapter. The focus is strictly on your ideas and the connections you make between academic content and personal experiences. You can also use the personal pronoun *I* in journal writing.

Checklist

Cultural Influences on Nursing Practice

_____ Definition of culture is appropriate.

_____ Importance of cultural competence in nursing is discussed.

_____ Discussion of <u>three</u> ways in which culture influences nursing, including specific examples, is thoughtful and thorough.

_____ Appropriate material from 4–5 outside sources (including paraphrasing and selective quoting; formatting of quotes; effective integration of quotes into paper) is integrated.

_____ Documentation of outside sources into body of paper (in-text citations) is accurate.

_____ Discussion of ways your cultural background may influence you as a nurse, including examples, is thoughtful and thorough.

_____ Style of writing is <u>concise</u> (no unnecessary words, no redundancy or repetition), <u>precise</u> (exact in meaning), and <u>clear</u>.

_____ Paper is well-organized: <u>introduction</u> includes definitions of culture and cultural competence and thesis statement; <u>logical order</u> of ideas in body exists; use of <u>transitions</u> between main points and parts of paper is appropriate; <u>conclusion</u> ties discussion of your cultural background to discussion of how culture influences nursing.

_____ Reference list is thorough (all in-text citations are in reference list and vice versa).

_____ Reference list is complete and accurate, using APA format.

_____ There are few, if any, errors in grammar, spelling, and punctuation.

_____ Revision reflects careful attention to instructor and peer feedback.

UNIT

4

Developing Note-Taking Skills for Nursing

The **content-based objective** includes understanding the role of culture in terms of the perception of and response to mental illness.

The **skill-based objectives** include

- Effective listening
- Understanding the various note-taking systems: guided notes/outline, think-link, Cornell.
- Note-taking strategies and skills: listening for signal words and phrases, recognizing repetition and redundancy, using telegraphic language, using symbols and abbreviations, recognizing stress and intonation

At the end of the unit, you will reflect on your understanding and attitude toward mental health and illness and any difficulties you anticipate as a nurse working with mentally ill patients.

Why Listening?

Many nursing courses rely heavily on lectures to deliver course content. Your ability to listen and take notes effectively is essential to doing well in those courses. In this unit, you will work on your listening and note-taking skills while exploring the topic of mental health and illness, an area of health care that can be challenging for students from cultures that may understand and respond to mental illness in ways that are very different from the United States.

Pre-Listening Activities

Before you listen to the lecture on mental health and illness, you will discuss mental illness from a cultural perspective and read articles that discuss mental illness from different cultural perspectives.

Discuss your answers to the questions. Form groups with classmates who do not have the same cultural background.

1. What do you know about mental illness?
2. Do you know someone who has been mentally ill? Describe the illness and how others responded to that person. If you don't know anyone, imagine how others might treat someone with a mental illness.
3. In your culture, what do people tend to think causes mental illness? How is it treated? Do you agree? Why or why not?
4. What are your concerns, as a nurse, about working with mentally ill patients?

The National Alliance on Mental Illness (NAMI) defines mental illness as "medical conditions that disrupt a person's thinking, feeling, mood, ability to relate to others, and daily functioning" (2007, para 1).

Readings about Mental Illness

Cultures have very different beliefs about what causes mental illness and how it should be treated. These beliefs can sometimes be at odds with how mental illness is understood and treated in the U.S. health care system.

The two readings discuss beliefs and practices for mental illness in Vietnamese and Liberian cultures. As you read these articles, think about similarities between what is presented and the beliefs and practices in your native culture.

Reading 4.1

Mental Health and Illness in Vietnamese Refugees

Steven Gold, PhD, Whittier, California,
Department of Sociology, Whittier College

Despite their impressive progress in adapting to American life, many Vietnamese still suffer from wartime experiences, culture shock, the loss of loved ones, and economic hardship. Although this ***trauma*** *creates substantial mental health needs, culture, experience, and the complexity of the American resettlement system often block obtaining assistance. Vietnamese mental health needs are best understood in terms of the family unit, which is extended, collectivistic, and patriarchal. Many refugees suffer from broken family status. They also experience role reversals wherein the increased social and economic power of women and children (versus men and adults) disrupts the traditional family ethos. Finally, cultural conflicts often make communication between practitioners and clients difficult and obscure central issues in mental health treatment. Rather than treating symptoms alone, mental health workers should acknowledge the cultural, familial, and historical context of Vietnamese refugees.*

A recently arrived Vietnamese woman who believed she was taken over by a ghost was brought by family members to the Community Mental Health Agency. Our staff was unable to help her. After a period of time, she asked us to take her to a Buddhist Temple. We did. She was exorcised and prayed over. After that, she was fine.

In retrospect, we have many questions. What really happened? Is this an appropriate **modality** of treatment? Can we bridge between the client and an outside source of assistance or are we legitimizing a method of treatment that is totally unscientific but may work?

Incident reported by Medical Social Worker in San Francisco, CA

More than 700,000 Vietnamese currently live in the United States. By century's end, they will be the third largest Asian-American group.[1] They are a socially diverse population whose members range from Western-educated professionals to rural peasants. Although the Vietnamese have made impressive progress in adjusting to life in the United States, many still suffer from various difficulties rooted in wartime experiences, their flight from home, culture shock, racial prejudice, the loss of and separation from loved ones, and economic hardship. As indicated in the story, addressing these issues offers unique challenges for mental health professionals. In this article I outline the resettlement experience of Vietnamese refugees and describe their efforts to obtain mental health services in the United States.

---

[1]Gardner, R.W., Robey, B., & Smith, P. C. (1985). Asian Americans: Growth, change and diversity. *Population Bulletin*, 40–51.

Flight and Adjustment for Three Subgroups

The Vietnamese refugee population is made up of three distinct subgroups—the first-wave elite, the boat people, and the ethnic Chinese. These three groups share a common experience as refugees, with similar cultural values and frequent interaction, but they also retain many social and cultural differences and have developed fairly disparate patterns of adaptation to the United States. Accordingly, their mental health needs and ways of relating to professional helpers are frequently distinct.

The first group of Vietnamese refugees entered the United States between 1975 and 1977. As former U.S. employees and members of the South Vietnamese military and government elite, many arrived with families intact. Their links to Western culture are indicated by their high levels of formal education and the fact that almost half were Catholic, even though more than 80 percent of all Vietnamese are Buddhists.[2, 3] Drawing on their skills, education, competence in English, familiarity with Western culture, and extended families, many adjusted rapidly. By the mid-1980s, the Office of Refugee Resettlement reported that the average income of first-wave refugees matched that of the larger U.S. population.[4]

The second wave of Vietnamese refugees—commonly called the boat people—began to enter the United States after the outbreak of the Vietnam-China conflict of 1978. Generally hailing from more plebeian origins and characterized by less education and lower levels of English competence than the first wave, these refugees lived for three or more years under Communism, sometimes laboring in re-education camps or remote "new economic zones" before leaving Vietnam. Their exit, involving clandestine escapes and open-sea voyages in leaky, overcrowded boats or long journeys on foot across revolution-torn Cambodia to Thailand, was subject to attack by pirates and military forces. Reportedly as many as half of those who attempted such an escape from Vietnam perished in flight. Those lucky enough to survive spent several months in the overcrowded refugee camps of Thailand, Malaysia, Indonesia, the Philippines, or Hong Kong before entering the United States.[5]

Owing to the dangers of escape, far more young men than women, children, or older people left Vietnam as boat people, yielding broken families and imbalanced sex ratios.[6] The boat people had more severe troubles in adapting economically than earlier arriving Vietnamese—including high levels of unemployment and welfare dependency (64 percent) and low rates of labor force participation (37 percent, more than 1 1/2 times the national average). Thousands continue to live below the poverty level (Table 1).[7, 8]

Within the second cohort of Vietnamese refugees, a sizable subpopulation exists. This group comprises members of Vietnam's ethnic Chinese minority, most of whom arrived after 1978 as boat people. Constituting an entrepreneurial class, these refugees frequently create Chinese-Vietnamese organizations and businesses in the United States. Because of ethnic differences and economic conflicts with the ethnic Vietnamese, relations between Chinese-Vietnamese and eth-

---

[2]Kelly, G. P. (1977). *From Vietnam to America: A chronicle of the Vietnamese immigration to the United States*. Boulder, CO: Westview Press.

[3]Hickey, G. C. (1964). *Village in Vietnam*. New Haven, CT: Yale University Press.

[4]Report to Congress: Refugee Resettlement Program. (1989). Washington, DC: Office of Refugee Resettlement.

[5]Teitelbaum, M. S. (1985). Forced migration: The tragedy of mass expulsion. In N. Glazer (Ed.), *Clamor at the gates: The New American immigration* (pp. 261–283). San Francisco: Institute for Contemporary Studies.

[6]Balvanz, B. (1988). Determination of the number of Southeast Asian refugee births and pregnancies by California county. *Migrant World, 16*, 7–16.

[7]Report to Congress: Refugee Resettlement Program. (1983). Washington, DC: Office of Refugee Resettlement.

[8]Rumbaut, R. G. (1989). The structure of refuge: Southeast Asian refugees in the United States, 1975–1985. *International Review of Comparative Public Policy, 1*, 97–129.

Table 1 Characteristics of Vietnamese Refugees in the United States: First Wave and Boat People*

	Vietnamese Refugees	
Characteristic	**First Wave (1975–1977)**	**Boat People (1978 and after)**
Average years of education	9.5	7.05
No English on arrival, %	30.6	50
Age		
% <36 yr	30.6	58
% >56 yr	10	5
White collar occupation		
in Vietnam, %	78.7	49.2
1980 Household income		
<$9,000, %	27.6	61
>$21,000, %	31	4.6

*From Office of Refugee Resettlement[9] and Nguyen and Henkin.[10]

nic Vietnamese were often strained in the country of origin, and many of these conflicts continue in the U.S.[10, 11]

Because few Chinese-Vietnamese have a Western education, they seldom work as high-level professionals, such as resettlement workers or Western health care professionals. Many are **practitioners** of Chinese traditional medicine, however. The existing network of refugee professionals and agencies that provides services to the refugee community is staffed by the ethnic Vietnamese, a group that many Chinese-Vietnamese consider hostile, making them reluctant to use such services. Health care professionals need to be aware of such interethnic conflicts when dealing with clients and supervising refugee staff.[13, 14, 15]

---

[9]Report to Congress.
[10]Nguyen, L. T., & Henkin, A. (1984). Vietnamese refugees in the United States: Adaptation and transitional status. *Journal of Ethnic Studies, 9,* 110–116.
[11]Gold, S. J. (1992). *Refugee communities: A comparative field study.* Newbury Park, CA: Sage.
[12]Peters, H., Schieffelin, B., Sexton, L., & Feingold, D. (1983). Who are the Sino-Vietnamese? *Culture, ethnicity and social categories: ORR Report.* Philadelphia, PA: Institute for the Study of Human Issues.
[13]Rumbaut, The structure of refuge.
[14]Desbarats, J. (1986). Ethnic differences in adaptation: Sino-Vietnamese refugees in the United States. *International Migration Review, 20,* 405–427.
[15]Westermeyer, J. (1990). Working with an interpreter in psychiatric assessment and treatment. *Journal of Nervous & Mental Diseases, 178,* 745–749.

Family Issues among Recently Arrived Vietnamese

The traditional Vietnamese family is perhaps the most basic, enduring, and self-consciously acknowledged form of national culture among refugees. It is customarily a large, **patriarchal,** and **extended** unit including minor children, married sons, daughters-in-law, unmarried grown daughters, and grandchildren under the same roof. **Individualism** is discouraged, whereas **collective** obligations and decision making are emphasized.[16] The traditional family has been altered as a consequence of Western influence, urbanization, and the war-**induced** absence of men. Nevertheless, many Vietnamese continue to uphold this social form as the preferable basis of social organization in the United States.

Positive adaptation is often facilitated through family-based cooperation.[17–21] Because of wartime casualties and tenuous condition of escape, however, many Vietnamese refugees must contend with broken families in the U.S. This, combined with cultural factors, such as the American emphasis on **nuclear** families, makes family adjustment **traumatic** for many Vietnamese. Prizing family connections, groups of recently arrived unattached male refugees create **"pseudofamilies"**—households made up of close and distant relatives and friends.[22] Sharing accommodations, finances, and fellowship, these collectives form an important source of social support in the refugee community. Although refugees find some comfort in household networks, their ability to establish regular families is often limited by poor economic status and the scarcity of Vietnamese women in the United States.[23,24]

Role Reversals

Vietnamese refugees of all subgroups have various degrees of reversal of the "provider" and "recipient" roles that existed among family members in Vietnam.[25] A common shift of roles occurs between husband and wife, with the wife taking on the breadwinner role and some of the status and power that accompany it. This is because women's jobs—hotel maid, sewing machine operator, and food service worker—are more readily available than the male-oriented unskilled occupations that the husband seeks. In other cases the wife becomes the breadwinner and supports the family by working in a menial job while the husband attempts to find professional employment. Finally, some women have to assume breadwinner roles because of the absence of a spouse in the U.S. Role changes also occur in families where both the husband and wife work because the wife was generally not employed outside the home before the family came to this country.

Role reversals between parents and children are also common because children often learn the English language and American customs rapidly and may be able to find employment more quickly than older members of the family. Such role reversals often yield **generational conflicts** within

---

[16]Henkin, A. B., & Nguyen, L. T. (1986). *Between two cultures: The Vietnamese in America.* Saratoga, CA: Century Twenty One Publishing.

[17]Gold, S. J. (1989). Differential adjustment among new immigrant family members. *Journal of Contemporary Ethnography, 17,* 408–434.

[18]Kibria, N. (1989). Patterns of Vietnamese refugee women's wagework in the U.S. *Ethnic Groups, 7,* 297–323.

[19]Kibria, N. (1990). Power, patriarchy, and gender conflict in the Vietnamese immigrant community. *Gender & Society, 4,* 9–24.

[20]Haines, D., Rutherford, D., & Thomas, P. (1981). Family and community among Vietnamese refugees. *International Migration Review, 15,* 310–319.

[21]Caplan, N., Whitmore, J. K., & Choy, M. H. (1989). *The boat people and achievement in America: A study of family life, hard work and cultural values.* Ann Arbor, MI: University of Michigan Press.

[22]Owan, T. C. (1985). Southeast Asian mental health: Transition from treatment services to prevention—A new direction. In T. C. Owan (Ed.), *Southeast Asian mental health: Treatment, prevention, services, training and research (pp. 141–167).* Washington, DC: U.S. Dept of Health and Human Services (DHHS).

[23]Gordon, L. W. (1982). *New data on the fertility of Southeast Asian Refugees in the U.S.* Paper presented at the Annual Meeting of the Population Association of America, San Diego, CA.

[24]Gordon, L. W. (1987). *The missing children: Mortality and fertility in a Southeast Asian refugee population.* Paper presented at the Annual Meeting of the Population Association of America, Chicago, IL.

[25]Sluzki, C. E. (1979). Migration and family conflict. *Family Process, 18,* 381–394.

refugee families in which the traditional culture is **collectivistic** and emphasizes the **deferential** treatment of elders, whereas American society is **individualistic** and youth oriented.[26] For young refugees, the pressure to conform simultaneously to American and Vietnamese cultures—which are in many ways **incompatible**—is a major source of strain.

Since the late 1980s, thousands of survivors of re-education camps, mostly former government and military officials and nearly all ethnic Vietnamese men, have been permitted to leave Vietnam and join their families who are already well established in the United States. These families are especially **susceptible** to traumatic **role reversals** and other family troubles because of the long period of separation. Further, although the husband may wish to retake his role as breadwinner and **patriarch,** he is ill-equipped to accomplish this task because he is unaccustomed to American society and must overcome the effects of years of incarceration.[27]

The process by which women or children rather than men become the primary source of refugee family income indicates the **adaptability** of Vietnamese families. At the same time, however, the inversion of traditional family roles often provokes hostility and resentment. Social workers with refugee clients comment that self-destructive, violent, **psychosomatic,** or antisocial reactions—such as wife or child abuse, depression, or alcoholism—occur as a result of family role reversals.[28–31] Role reversals are especially traumatic for the Chinese-Vietnamese because they often maintain more traditional family patterns than the ethnic Vietnamese.[32]

Media reports and academic research reveal—and often overemphasize—the **bipolar adaptation** of Vietnamese youth. One group, most often children of first-wave refugees, are "academic superstars," graduating first in their class at many top schools and colleges including the U.S. Naval Academy.[33,34] At the other end of the social spectrum is the involvement of Vietnamese youth in various criminal and gang activities, which are often directed toward other Asian immigrants.[35] Although these two groups illustrate the diversity of Vietnamese adaptation, most refugee youth fall somewhere between the sensationalized polarities of superachiever and delinquent.

Refugee Resettlement System

Vietnamese refugees in the United States must weave through a complex maze of agencies to address the social, economic, and adjustment problems they experience. In so doing they find that their indigenous approaches to problem solving, authority relations, and helping relationships are different from the outlook maintained by the institutions and staff of the resettlement system.[36,37]

---

[26]Brower, I. (1981). Counseling Vietnamese. In *Bridging cultures: Southeast Asian refugees in America*, (pp. 224–240). Los Angeles: Asian American Community Mental Health Training Center.

[27]*Report to Congress: Refugee Resettlement Program.* (1990). Washington, DC: Office of Refugee Resettlement.

[28]Cohon, J. D., Jr. (1981). Psychological adaptation and dysfunction among refugees. *International Migration Review, 15,* 255–275.

[29]Portes, A., & Rumbaut, R.G. (1990). *Immigration America: A portrait.* Berkeley, CA: University of California Press.

[30]Chan, K. B., & Lam, L. (1987). Psychological problems of Chinese Vietnamese refugees resettling in Quebec. In K.B. Chan & D.M. Indra (Eds.), *Uprooting, loss and adaptation: The Resettlement of Indochinese refugees in Canada* (pp. 27–41). Ottawa, Canadian Public Health Association.

[31]Takaki, R. (1989). *Strangers from a different shore: A history of Asian Americans.* Boston: Little, Brown.

[32]Chan, K. B., & Lam, L. (1987). Community, kinship and family in the Chinese Vietnamese community: Some enduring values and patterns of interaction. In K. B. Chan & D. M. Indra (Eds.), *Uprooting, loss and adaptation: The resettlement of Indochinese refugees in Canada* (pp. 15–26). Ottawa: Canadian Public Health Association.

[33]Caplan et al., *The boat people.*

[34]Takaki, *Strangers from a different shore.*

[35]Vigil, J. D., & Yun S. C. (1990). Vietnamese youth gangs in Southern California. In R. Huff (Ed.), *Gangs in America* (pp. 146–162). Newbury Park, CA: Sage.

[36]de Voe, D. M. (1981). Framing refugees as clients. *International Migration Review, 15,* 88–94.

[37]Williams, C. L. (1987). *Prevention programs for refugees: An interface for mental health and public health.* Rockville, MD: National Institute of Mental Health, Contract No. 278-85-0024 CH.

Resettlement and refugee-aid services are delivered and administered by a diverse network of government, religious, nonprofit, and profit-making agencies and organizations. For example, in 1983, there were over 40 agencies resettling Vietnamese refugees in San Francisco alone, with 15 or more in surrounding counties.[38] The large number of resettlement agencies providing service to Vietnamese refugees was inefficient in terms of coordination and allocation of funding and sometimes created interagency competition and hostility.[39–41]

A major role in the resettlement of refugees is carried out by 13 voluntary agencies funded by the federal government.[42] These agencies are decentralized, often overlapping, have few professional staff, and are subject to severe fiscal problems. They generally provide only short-term and survival-type aid. Because most are directed specifically toward the problems of Southeast Asian refugees, few existed before 1975. Further, after the peak of migration in the early 1980s, many agencies had heavy cutbacks in staff and funding or were phased out altogether.

Refugees have a hard time locating agencies that are capable of helping them. A Washington State study revealed that between 50 percent and 70 percent of refugees did not know how to obtain vital services such as legal help, free emergency medical care, English classes, free emergency food, or low-income housing that were available to them.[43] Refugees who do use services tend to be among the elite of the community—the 1975 cohort.[44] Refugee clients generally find word-of-mouth referrals from trusted peers to be the most useful source of information about helping agencies.

Interactions with Treatment Staff

Interactions with agency staff and helping professionals frequently take place in an environment of distorted communication and cultural **incompatibility**.[45] These misunderstandings become painfully apparent when refugees seek mental health assistance. Health **assessments** show that refugees suffer from various mental health problems that are far more severe than those of **voluntary immigrants** and the native born.[46] Those most frequently reported are major **depressive disorders, schizophrenia,** and anxiety and other **neurotic** conditions.[47, 48–50] Vietnamese refugees also suffer from medical problems. Consequently, federal, state, and local governments have funded a number of mental health programs for this population.[51,52]

---

[38]Murray, M., & Associates. (1981). *A report on refugee services in San Francisco.* San Francisco: Center for Southeast Asian Refugee Resettlement.

[39]Gold, S. J. (1987). Dealing with frustration: A study of interactions between resettlement staff and refugees. In S. Morgan & E. Colson (Eds.), *People in upheaval* (pp. 108–128). New York: Center for Migration Studies.

[40]Finnan, C. R., & Cooperstein, R. *Southeast Asian refugee resettlement at the local level.* Menlo Park, CA: SRI International.

[41]*State plan for refugee assistance and services, federal fiscal year 1983.* (1982). Sacramento, CA: State Dept of Social Services, Office of Refugee Services.

[42]*Report to Congress: Refugee resettlement program.* (1984). Washington, DC: Office of Refugee Resettlement.

[43]Wilson, W. L., & Garrick, M. A. *Refugee assistance termination study.* Olympia, WA: State Dept. of Social and Health Services.

[44]Caplan, N., Whitmore J. K., & Bui, Q. L. (1985). *Southeast Asian refugee self-sufficiency study: ORR report.* Ann Arbor, MI: The Institute for Social Research, University of Michigan.

[45]*Assessment of the MAA incentive grant initiative—ORR report.* (1986). Washington, DC: Lewin & Associates.

[46]Vega, W. A. & Rumbaut, R. G. (1991). Ethnic minorities and mental health. *Annual Review of Sociology, 17,* 351–383.

[47]Brower, I. (1981). Counseling Vietnamese. In *Bridging cultures: Southeast Asian refugees in America* (pp. 224–240), Los Angeles: Asian American Community Mental Health Training Center.

[48]Kinzie, J. D. (1985). Overview of clinical issues in the treatment of Southeast Asian refugees. In T. C. Owan (Ed.), Southeast Asian mental health: *Treatment, prevention, services, training and research* (pp. 113–134). Washington, DC: US DHHS.

[49]Young, R. F., Bukoff, A., Waller, J. B. Jr., & Blount, S. B. (1987). Health status, health problems and practices among refugees from the Middle East, Eastern Europe and Southeast Asia. *International Migration Review, 21,* 760–782.

[50]Ishisaka, H. A., Nguyen, Q. T., & Okimoto, J. T. (1985). The role of culture in the mental health treatment of Indochinese refugees. In T. C. Owan (Ed.), *Southeast Asian mental health: Treatment, prevention, services, training and research* (pp. 41–63). Washington, DC: US DHHS.

[51]Lappin, J. & Scott, S. (1982). Intervention in a Vietnamese refugee family. In M. McGoldrick, J. K. Pearce & J. Giordano (Eds.), *Ethnicity and family therapy* (pp. 483–491). New York: Guilford Press.

[52]Cichon, D. J., Gozdziak, E. M., & Grover, J. G. (1986). *The economic and social adjustment of non-southeast Asian refugees—*Vol I, *Analysis across cases: ORR report.* Dover, NH: Research Management Corp.

Unfortunately, most Vietnamese lack the cultural prerequisites of a successful American-style **therapy** interaction, such as a willingness to confide, a belief in the unconscious, and the ability to criticize parents openly. They have limited familiarity with the treatment of **chronic** health problems and regard Western medication with a combination of awe and fear. There is no equivalent word in the Vietnamese language for the term **"counselor."** Mental health problems are so highly **stigmatized** by the Vietnamese that it is difficult even to discuss these issues without **provoking** feelings of shame. For example, even highly educated long-established refugees use the terms "mental health" and "mental illness" interchangeably.[53] Most refugees do not see a connection between the process of therapy and the problems that for them are most pressing.[54,55] According to Kinzie, "Many Southeast Asians have an unwillingness or an inability to differentiate between psychological, physiological, and **supernatural** causes of illness."[56] (p. 116).

Finally, because of their experience as refugees, Vietnamese do not easily trust authority figures, including treatment staff. Accordingly, refugees often avoid seeking help until the situation is intolerable, and when they do, cooperative relations between helpers and clients are extremely difficult to establish. A Vietnam-born American-educated director of a refugee mental health program described his relations with clients as follows: "For an average Vietnamese, mental health would immediately mean that the person is crazy, acting crazy, saying crazy things."

As a consequence of refugees' difficulties in gaining access to helping agencies and because of their general reluctance to contact professionals to resolve mental health problems, few Vietnamese clients **voluntarily** seek mental health assistance. Most are referred to service providers by schools, the criminal justice system, and other agencies. Those who willingly seek professional help have often reached a level of desperation. Self-referred clients are generally one of two types. The first type contacts the agency not because of emotional problems but because of practical difficulties, which are often financial in nature—lack of basic necessities such as food, housing, a job, and child care—and the client has no other resource. This type of client comes to the agency out of desperation. Survival problems have become more common recently because of bad economic times and cutbacks in social service programs. Because of confusion in culture and communication, however, discovering the fact that clients' needs, however serious, are rooted in environmental rather than **psychiatric** difficulties often takes considerable time and effort, even with Vietnamese-speaking staff.

The second category of self-referred clients is those who are having **acute** mental health difficulties that family members or the affected person can no longer manage. As Muecke has noted,

> "**Disturbed** persons are usually harbored within their family unless they become destructive, at which point they may be admitted to hospital . . . or otherwise **restrained,** but at the great cost of bringing shame to the family."[57] (p. 34)

Through mutual misunderstandings, helping professionals and refugee clients often unwittingly engage in a "conspiracy of silence" that prevents direct confrontation of the problems at hand. This is further exacerbated by both parties' attempts to avoid embarrassment. Treatment staff resist asking specific questions about mental health problems, and refugees fail to **volunteer** relevant

---

[53]Wong, J. (1981). Appropriate mental health treatment and service delivery systems for Southeast Asians. In *Bridging cultures: South Asian refugees in America* (pp. 195–224). Los Angeles, CA: Asian American Community Mental Health Training Center.

[54]Beiser, M. (1991). The mental health of refugees in resettlement countries, In H. Adelman (Ed.), *Refugee policy: Canada and the United States* (pp. 425–442). Toronto: York Lanes Press.

[55]Rumbaut, R. G. (1991). Migration, adaptation and mental health: The experience of Southeast Asian refugees in the United States. In H. Adelman (Ed.), *Refugee policy: Canada and the United States.* (pp. 381–424). Toronto: York Lanes Press.

[56]Kinzie, Overview of clinical issues.

[57]Muecke, M. A. (1983). In search of healers—Southeast Asian refugees in the American health care system. *The Western Journal of Medicine, 139,* 835–840 [31–36].

information. After finally identifying the source of a problem, a physician will state, "Why didn't you tell me?" to which the patient replies, "You didn't ask me."

Practical Suggestions for Clinicians

Practitioners familiar with Vietnamese clients recommend a variety of strategies for addressing the problems of Vietnamese refugee clients. The most general theme might be called a global approach. To untangle the nature of the clients' problems, clinicians need to know about their personal histories, including life in Vietnam, the experience of flight, stay in the refugee camp, and the nature of their current circumstances in the U.S., such as family, job, and health status.[58–61] Because refugees may suffer from physical health problems and frequently **somatize** mental health issues, treatment staff should have access to clients' medical evaluations.[62]

Because refugees are embarrassed by mental health concerns, practitioners should approach such matters in a straightforward manner. This can be fostered by obtaining background information about patients. When mentioned strategically, such information encourages clients to abandon their efforts to maintain a false front that "everything is okay."[63] For similar reasons treatment staff are encouraged to ask their patients direct and specific questions about symptoms. The general question, "How do you feel?" as asked by American physicians is all but meaningless to Vietnamese patients. Instead, the question should be, "How do you hurt?" or "Where does it hurt?"

Treatment staff need to be able to distinguish between mental health problems shaped by culture and those caused by life experiences. For example, although culturally sensitive mental health workers often assume that Vietnamese patients suffer from depression, passivity, interpersonal problems, **somatization,** and unemployment because of culture shock and the effects of "the Asian worldview," these symptoms may actually have their origins in war-induced **posttraumatic stress disorder,** a **syndrome** common to American Vietnam veterans.[64]

As refugees, many Vietnamese have adopted a survival-oriented approach to life. They are more likely to perceive physical symptoms and concrete needs as crucial sources of difficulty. Emotional or psychological problems are seen as less serious or immediate. Although this often serves as an obstacle to treatment, it is also a possible source of strength. Helpers are encouraged to remind refugee clients of their abilities used to overcome past personal challenges and to rely on these coping abilities to resolve contemporary concerns. Selective inclusion of past experiences is also suggested as an important element in therapy so that clients do not ignore traumatic experiences, dwell excessively on painful incidents, or long nostalgically for an idealized past.[65,66]

As a means of dealing with the **stigma** of mental health problems, Vietnamese refugees often indicate their symptoms by referring to physical problems. In helping refugees deal with physical and concrete matters, however, treatment staff can establish the trusting relations that are essential for addressing submerged psychological issues. Further, although Vietnamese are unfamiliar with

---

[58] Kinzie, Overview of clinical issues.

[59] Wong, Appropriate mental health treatment.

[60] August, L. & Gianola, B. A. (1987). Symptoms of war trauma induced psychiatric disorder: Southeast Asian refugees and Vietnam veterans. *International Migration Review, 21,* 820–832.

[61] Chan, K. B., & Loveridge, D. (1987). Refugees 'in transit': Vietnamese in a refugee camp in Hong Kong. *International Migration Review, 21,* 745–759.

[62] Kinzie, Overview of clinical issues.

[63] Ishisaka, et al., The role of culture.

[64] August & Gianola, Symptoms of war trauma.

[65] Chan & Lam, Psychological problems.

[66] Beiser, M. (1991). The mental health of refugees in resettlement countries, In H. Adelman (Ed.), *Refugee policy: Canada and the United States* (pp. 425–442). Toronto: York Lanes Press.

the role of a mental health counselor or **psychotherapist,** their cultural experience is **compatible** with that of the physician-patient relationship and sick role. Hence, **psychiatrists** are encouraged to consider prescribing medication to relieve symptoms. Accustomed to traditional Asian herbal medicine, refugees endow Western medications with mythic power. Such treatments impress refugees, but care providers nevertheless report **noncompliance,** with clients reducing or forgoing **doses** because of the **cessation** of symptoms, the occurrence of side effects, or the advice of family members. Blood tests are warranted to assess patient **compliance.**[67]

In helping refugees deal with adapting to the American culture, the bicultural approach is generally most appropriate. Refugees who have connections with indigenous traditions and coethnic communities as well as the cultural and linguistic skills required for interacting with the large society appear to achieve the highest levels of economic progress and emotional well-being.[68–70]

Finally, because of the central role of the family in Vietnamese life, health workers should understand that they are not only treating a person, but are also indirectly interacting with a group of **kin.** Treatment staff are advised to enlist the cooperation and trust of the family unit to avoid competitive relations with relatives that may become an obstacle to effective treatment. Because of patients' extensive involvement with their families, mental health professionals need to practice discretion rather than confidentiality in their interactions with family members.[71]

Conclusions

Vietnamese are a socially diverse group. Although their traumatic flight from home and resettlement in the United States often result in substantial mental health needs, their culture and experience make them wary of interactions with mental health workers.

To interact effectively with Vietnamese refugees, mental health workers need to approach them in a **holistic** manner—understanding that their needs are shaped by their unique familial and cultural background. Treatment staff are likely to achieve more satisfactory results if they relate to Vietnamese clients in terms of this complex than if they attempt to treat **isolated** symptoms.

---

[67]Kinzie, Overview of clinical issues.

[68]Chan & Lam, Community, kinship and family.

[69]Rumbaut, R. G. (1991). Migration, adaptation and mental health: The experience of Southeast Asian refugees in the United States. In H. Adelman (Ed.), *Refugee policy: Canada and the United States* (pp. 381–424). Toronto: York Lanes Press.

[70]Westermeyer, J., Callies, A., & Neider, J. (1990). Welfare status and psychosocial adjustment among 100 Hmong refugees. *Journal of Nervous & Mental Diseases, 178,* 300–306.

[71]Wong, Appropriate mental health treatment.

Activity: Vocabulary Development

Reading 4.1 contains many mental health and other specialized medical/ nursing terms and socio-cultural terms. Add the words you do not know to your dictionary, following the guidelines on page 33. Use a medical English dictionary to look up mental health and other specialized medical/ nursing terms and a college-level English dictionary to look up the socio-cultural terms that you do not know. Use 10–15 new words in answering the discussion questions.

Comprehension and Discussion Questions

The questions ask you to locate important information in the article, as well as think beyond what is stated in the reading—for example, by comparing and contrasting what you have learned about mental illness and the Vietnamese community to your own cultural community in the United States or to immigrant/refugee communities in general. In small groups, discuss your answers to these questions.

1. The article compares and contrasts traditional family structure in Vietnam and U.S. family structure. Fill in the chart with contrasting adjectives.

Families in Vietnam	**Families in the U.S.**
extended	____________________
____________________	individualistic
____________________	matriarchal*
deferential to elderly	____________________

2. Why have role reversals between husband and wife occurred in Vietnamese families in the United States? Why have they occurred between parents and children?
3. What are some of the negative effects of both kinds of role reversal?
4. Have role reversal and intergenerational conflict occurred in your cultural community in the United States? Why or why not?
5. In your opinion, what are some ways to prevent the negative effects of role reversals in your cultural community or immigrant/refugee communities in general?

**Note:* This word does not appear in the article, but it is the opposite of a word that does.

6. On page 130, the author states "refugees suffer from various mental health problems that are far more severe than those of voluntary immigrants and the native born." What are some differences between voluntary immigrants and refugees to the United States? Why do you think refugees experience greater problems with mental illness than voluntary immigrants?
7. Why is "American-style therapy," as described in the article (page 131), unlikely to work with Vietnamese clients? Do you think "American-style therapy" would work with clients from your cultural background? Why or why not?
8. Why is noncompliance with medication often a problem with Vietnamese clients? Do you think clients from your cultural background would stop taking medication without their doctor's approval? Why or why not?
9. Why are direct, specific questions like, "Where does it hurt?" (page 132) preferable to "How do you feel?" (page 132) with Vietnamese clients?
10. What other strategies does the author recommend for working successfully with Vietnamese clients? What other strategies would you recommend?

Reading 4.2

West African Beliefs about Mental Illness

Ann Hales, PhD, RN, Associate Professor, New Mexico State University, Las Cruces, NM

Mental health/psychiatric nurses are becoming more sensitized to the need for incorporating cultural data in the assessment and care of their clients (Tripp-Reimer & Lively, 1993). Indeed, understanding a client's cultural beliefs is a core value central to health care, the nursing profession, and nursing education (Leininger, 1970, 1978, 1985, 1993; Murillo-Rohde, 1978; Spector, 1985). Moreover, ignoring a client's cultural beliefs can seriously **compromise** quality nursing care, thereby limiting the client's return to a state of health (Leininger, 1978). Ideally, nursing educators ensure inclusion of cultural content in the nursing curricula. Cultural issues became relevant to me when faced with the task of teaching psychiatric nursing to Liberian nursing students from a cultural perspective entirely different from my own. For two years, I lived in Liberia, West Africa, while serving as a Peace Corps volunteer. As a nurse-educator from a different culture than both the students and clients, I explored Liberian beliefs regarding the causes and treatment of mental illness.

Ethnohistory

Liberia is a republic on the west coast of Africa. Located on the North Atlantic Ocean between Cote d'Ivoire and Sierra Leone, and bound by Guinea to its north, it is slightly larger than Tennessee. Thirty ethnic groups with 30 different languages reside within this area. The republic of Liberia was established in 1822 by the National Colonization Society of America. This society was founded to repatriate American slaves to Africa. In 1848, Liberian Governor Joseph Jenkins Roberts proclaimed Liberia an independent republic. Liberia was recognized by the United States as such in 1862.

The population of Liberia, estimated in 1993 to be 2.8 million is 95 percent indigenous and 5 percent descendants of repatriated U.S. slaves. Liberia's Western influences were brought by these black American settlers (repatriated slaves), rather than by white European colonists. Seventy percent of Liberians practice traditional religions; approximately 40 percent of the total population can read and write. The **life expectancy** of a Liberian male is 54.88 years, and 59.76 years for a female. The **fertility rate** per woman is 6.42 children, and the **infant mortality rate** is 115.9 deaths per 1,000 live births.

Liberia has West Africa's largest tropical rain forest. Hot and humid, the annual mean temperature is about 82 degrees Fahrenheit. Annual rainfall varies from 70 inches to 200 inches, with the heaviest rainfall along the coast. The terrain is mostly flat to rolling coastal plains, with low mountains in the northeast.

Since 1990, civil war has destroyed much of Liberia's economy, especially the infrastructure in and around the nation's capital, Monrovia. Approximately 750,000 Liberian refugees have fled to neighboring countries (Goldberg, 1995), while 150,000 have been killed. A United States Travel Advisory prohibits Americans from entering Liberia (GPO62-830cc: The Ongoing Civil War, 1992). Evacuation of remaining expatriots in Liberia began in April 1996 and is now considered to be a completed process.

Cultural Assessment

When Oyefeso (1994) surveyed 480 senior federal civil servants in Nigeria about their attitudes toward ex-mental clients, he found pervasive negative attitudes. Wondering whether Liberian beliefs would be similar, I assigned the Liberian psychiatric nursing students two projects: a) to write a short paper about their experience with someone they believed to be mentally ill; and b) to interview a grandparent, older relative, or village elder about their beliefs about mental illness.

Each student informed the interviewees that their responses would be seen by the student's instructor, and that information would be summarized and possibly published. Students did not include the name of the person interviewed to assure privacy, anonymity, and confidentiality. If the interviewee was not comfortable with the process, or did not give his/her verbal consent, students were advised not to proceed with the interview.

Fourteen students completed both assignments. After reading each paper I compiled a list of various themes. The papers were reread for content analysis and themes were identified, synthesized, and categorized.

Findings

Three major categories regarding the causes of mental illness were identified: (1) a punishment for wrongdoing, (2) the result of being "witched" by another person, and (3) an illness that is "passed down" through the family.

Punishment

The belief that "wrongdoings" can cause a person to become mentally ill was common. Wrongdoings could range from a minor infraction, such as eating a taboo food, to a major violation, such as murdering a relative. The seriousness of the mental illness was seen to reflect the seriousness of the wrongdoing.

Offending the **ancestral** spirits, gods, and goddesses was seen as another kind of wrongdoing that could cause mental illness. A frequently mentioned spirit was Mammie Water. Having a female upper body and a fish lower body, Mammie Water usually appears to individuals in their dreams. She tells them to "prove their devotion" by **sacrificing** the thing/person they most love, and that if they worship her she will reward them with money, gifts, and talents. If a person has a dream about Mammie Water, but decides not to comply with her request for worship, the dreamer must confess to a zoe in order to prevent Mammie Water from causing harm. The following are excerpts from students' papers about Mammie Water:

> Old Man Karwee called a witch doctor to find out the reason for his son's illness. The witch doctor reported that Mammie Water, with whom Karwee dealt to make him brilliant in school, caused him to "go off" because he went against her. Karwee asked his father to have the witch doctor drive Mammie Water from behind him [get away from him]. Old Lady told me the story of a woman in our village who had not had any children. Since she was the first wife of her husband, the other two wives never allowed her to have any peace of mind about being **barren.** To get away from their talk, and to relieve her frustration, she usually went to the river to fish. Standing at the water side, one day, she felt weak and decided to rest on the bank. She fell into a deep sleep and had a dream in which an old man came from the river to tell her she would become pregnant within three months, if she agreed to abide by two conditions. The conditions were that she and her child were never to eat fish or to play around any large body of water.
>
> Her dream came true: She became pregnant and bore a daughter. Because of her fear she always abided by the conditions. However, her daughter followed some of her friends to the river when she was about 10 years old, without her mother knowing. No one

> knows what happened at the river. When she arrived home she started to act very unusual. Her mother took her to a country zoe, who diagnosed her as having seen Mammie Water. To make a **sacrifice** of one white sheep and one white chicken at midnight at the riverside was the only cure. These sacrifices were made, but the daughter was never quite the same. Whenever she had a spell her family made sacrifices to Mammie Water to restore her to normal.

Mammie Water is not the only spirit who can be offended. Ancestors and other deceased relatives, when offended, can cause a person to become mentally ill as well. A pregnant or **postpartum** woman is reported to be particularly susceptible to spirits, which follow and make her mentally ill. One student wrote that a pregnant woman can protect herself by carrying a penknife in her clothes. The woman must touch the knife when she thinks a spirit is near and continue to do so even after her child is born. The belief is that early postpartum is when the spirit will come to the mother at night, and offer her gold, money, and gifts in exchange for her devotion to him. If she does not rid herself of this spirit by touching the knife, she will become mentally ill.

In addition to offending spirits, there are other wrongdoings that can cause mental illness. One student wrote:

> Now craziness can attack anyone of any age. Generally, the cause is either eating one's taboo, disobedience, trespassing to a sacred area, or stealing.

Being Witched

The belief that another person can "witch" or "put medicine on" an individual believed to have acted wrongly was common. To "witch" another person, the individual must go to the village zoe, pay a fee, make sacrifices, and wait for the zoe to "throw his sign." If family members of a mentally ill person believe their loved one is a victim of a sign they may go to whomever they believed initiated the sign and beg for their relative to be released. They, too, then must go to the zoe, pay fees, and make sacrifices such as goats, sheep, roosters, or rice.

Female adultery is a behavior that is thought to cause mental illness, either because of the "wrongdoing" involved or because the woman was witched by her spouse for revenge. Stealing is another "wrongdoing" that may result in mental illness because the theft's victim decides to "put a sign" on the thief. One student wrote:

> Mental illness due to stealing usually occurs because the victim had a quick temper and went to the zoe to have bad medicine sworn on the thief. If the victim had been considerate he first would ask the town crier to inform the villagers to have someone confess. If no one confessed, then the victim could throw bad medicine and the thief would go crazy.

Signs also can be thrown because of jealousy. A beautiful woman or a brilliant man could become mentally ill because others in the village went to the zoe to have a sign thrown on the person because they were jealous. The following is one student's account of how a young boy became mentally ill as the result of others' jealousy:

> One man in our village took mentally ill when he was a young boy. He was the son of a rich man with over 20 wives. The boy was the first son of the head wife and was his father's most loved. All the other wives were jealous and decided to witch him to get him mad. They took a piece of his clothes to a zoe who used the clothes and made the boy go mad.

However, going to a zoe to make someone become mentally ill also can cause that individual to become mentally ill. A student writes: "People will become crazy from trying to witch others if the other person's spirit is stronger than their own." She further explains:

> When a man goes to a zoe to put a sign on someone else, or to ask for special talents, the zoe will give him certain laws to follow. Some of the things that he might go to the zoe for include: (1) wanting to be clever in school; (2) wanting to be a good hunter; or (3) wanting to have a lot of women be attracted to him. The zoe will have the man make sacrifices and follow laws such as (1) don't look back here from your house, (2) don't talk to anyone for three days, or (3) don't drink or eat anything for a day. If he violates these laws, he will go crazy. If the man is asking the zoe for a huge talent or gift, the laws will be much harder, like sacrificing a favorite child or bringing a leopard to the zoe. If the zoe is asked to make medicine to kill someone, the person is given a certain period of time to warn the victim. If he does not find them in that time, he will become crazy.

"Down-the-Line"

Another cause of mental illness reported by the students was "down-the-line" or **inherited** mental illness. Inherited mental illness is believed to be passed through only the mother, since she is the one who gives birth to the child. Inherited mental illness also can result when an **ancestor** has been so offensive to the spirits that the whole family is punished with mental illness.

Students reported that some types of "down-the-line" mental illness can be prevented. The most common methods of prevention include: (1) taking the newborn to the zoe, who will give the baby **preventative** country medicine and "mark" his/her back, (2) wearing a charm around one's neck that keeps away the angry spirits and (3) avoiding swimming because the water is controlled by the spirits.

Many students wrote about a type of inherited mental illness called "open mole." Open mole clients generally present themselves at the general hospital with an herbal paste on their scalps where the **fontanels** join. The generally accepted belief is that people with excessive symptoms of anxiety have a congenital opening at the **junction** of their fontanels, which provides an entry for evil spirits.

According to some elders, when mentally ill individuals die, some of them are born again with the same mental illness into the same family. Reportedly, the illness generally is passed to the most beloved child, and rarely, if ever, is **curable**. Thus, mental illness is passed down from generation to generation.

Various elders disagreed about whether mental illness is **contagious.** While most of them believed that mental illness was not contagious, they still believed the mentally ill should be avoided. The rationale was that a man who had committed an offense grave enough to cause his own mental illness certainly had angered the gods. To associate with such a man would invite the wrath of the gods and cause one's own mental illness.

The second aspect of the students' assignment was to interview elders concerning their beliefs about treatments of the mental illness. Paralleling the causes of mental illness, treatments also clustered into three categories, which included: (1) **confession** of wrongdoing, (2) removal of a spirit or the "thrown sign" through country medicine, and (3) prevention of "down-the-line" illness.

Confession, Sacrifice, and Cleansing

If a person's mental illness is believed to result from a wrongdoing, the first stage of the cure is to make a confession. Then, the ill person and his/her family make sacrifices to the person, or spirit, to whom the wrongdoing was done. The village zoe determines what sacrifices are required, as well as the fees due. Kola nuts, white chickens, roosters, and sheep are thought to be appropriate sacrifices. The average fee for service ranged between $5 and $25, but a fee of $150 was required for a particularly serious mental illness. After the individual **confesses** to his/her violation and sacrifices are made, a cleansing or **purification ritual** occurs.

Driving Out the Spirits

If a mental illness is believed to be caused by a spirit, treatment requires driving away those spirits by making sacrifices that satisfy the spirit, or by creating physical discomfort within the victim's body so the spirit will want to flee. Beating the victim is the most common method of driving out the evil spirit.

A mentally ill person often is subjected to purification **ceremonies** as well. In one ceremony a woman was placed in a steaming hut for two days; at the end of the second day the hut was set on fire. It is believed that if she is able to run out of the hut, then the spirit leaves her body and runs the other way. If, however, she cannot flee, the spirit is destroyed (along with the person). One elder considered this method of purification "too risky" and preferred an herbal purification treatment.

This elder would crush his herbs with **snuff** or mix it in fermented cane juice (an alcoholic beverage commonly drunk in Liberia). The herbal mixture then was placed in all **orifices** of the victim, i.e., nose, mouth, rectum, and even ears and eyes because spirits are thought to enter the individual via the body openings. The victim reportedly "becomes fierce" (violent) when the herbs are administered because evil spirits and the person are fighting. After about a week of this treatment, which frequently causes sneezing, vomiting, and diarrhea, the victim supposedly is cured. If a person is visually **hallucinating,** additional herbs are placed in his eyes so the things he sees will "come off."

Less traumatic purification ceremonies include the practice of writing "magic" words with chalk on a wooden plank. The plank is then washed with fresh water, which is used for drinking and bathing the victim.

"Down-the-Line" Treatment

If a person is mentally ill as the result of **heredity,** the treatment often is quite vigorous. One student reported on the treatment of a child who was believed to be mentally ill as the result of his mother's wrongdoing:

> A special kind of leaf was gathered from the bush and placed in his nostrils three times a day for a week. This caused him to vomit the bad substance that was passed to him through his mother's pregnancy. A large, very hot blanket was placed over his head to make him sweat out the evil spirits from his blood. At the end of the week the child was marched through the town in a ceremony. At the climax of the ceremony a live white chicken was buried and the gods were begged for forgiveness for the child's mother's wrongdoing.

Most "down-the-line" mental illnesses are seen as **incurable** based on the reasoning that the gods are so angry that they will not forgive the victim even after sacrifices have been made. Consequently, the ill person may be tied to a log in the bush or even left to die. One account of such an incidence follows:

> After a group of men catches them, they carry these people far into the bush to be treated with country medicine. A hole is dug in a tree that has been cut down. The person's feet are put in the hole and tied together tightly so he/she won't run away and cause trouble. Their clothes are taken off so that they won't hurt themselves. A small hut is built around the tree for shelter. A family member is left with the person to keep watch and a country doctor is present to treat the person. As they come back to their senses, they notice

> their clothes are off, their feet are tied, and they are in a strange area. They are given their clothes and set free to walk about.

If, for some reason, an incurable man is allowed to wander through the village, villagers will throw him food and water in an effort to keep him at a distance. Individuals also may be kept at a distance through brute force, such as rock throwing.

Implications for Nursing Practice and Education

After collecting information from the students about mental illness in Liberia, the challenge became to integrate this information with classroom and clinical teaching. The overwhelming majority of students who had encountered a mentally ill person had been extremely frightened of the person, believing that all mentally ill people were violent. One student reported:

> My mother was standing on the porch when she saw a young fellow coming toward her. Having heard about him, she went in the house for a knife, a fufu stick, and an empty beer bottle. When she returned, Beneto was standing on the porch waiting to attack her. When he saw that she was carrying a knife, stick, and bottle, he ran away. I think this is the best way to act when a mentally ill person comes near you. Don't allow him to know that you are afraid, or you will find yourself seriously damaged.

The student never indicated how her mother knew the ill man was "waiting to attack her," or stopped to wonder if her mother's defensive stance might have been unnecessary.

In the village where I lived I observed a group of approximately 20 children tease, harass, and throw pebbles at a man who was considered "not of sound mind." The children's final point of elation came when the man finally, after a great deal of tolerance of the children, picked up a handful of pebbles and scattered them at the children. As soon as the man responded by throwing the pebbles, the children stopped their teasing and became interested in other activity. One student who had observed similar situations concluded: "Mentally ill people are considered to be the center of amusement for children."

I realized the classroom could not function as the only arena for combating such beliefs about mental illness. The students and I lived on the psychiatric hospital grounds for a five-week clinical rotation in close association with the patients. Each morning and evening everyone met at a common well to draw their daily water. At these times, I always acknowledged and spoke with the patients, and came to know them quite well. This willingness to approach and talk with a patient became a beginning point for students to do the same. After the first week at the hospital, students approached patients more willingly and gradually some of their fear began to subside.

Although I learned that there were many differences between my own cultural beliefs and Liberian beliefs, rather than emphasizing differences, I sought some common ground. The following similarities between Liberian beliefs/practices and Western theory were identified:

a. The concept of guilt plays a role in the cause of mental illnesses in both perspectives. Guilt about one's "wrongdoing," rather than a spirit's response to the wrongdoing, could be a contributing factor in causing mental illness. Just as "confession" to a **therapist** provides relief in our Western culture, confession to a zoe might well have a similar outcome. That is, helping clients to talk about their feelings could serve a similar function as to what occurred when they visited a zoe and confessed their wrongdoing.

b. Holistic nursing in Western culture includes the belief that the therapeutic nurse-client relationship occurs when the client trusts the nurse and believes in the **therapeutic** process of the relationship, and accounts, in part, for some of the healing that occurs. Again, the therapeutic process was framed as having a similar function as visiting a zoe.

c. A person with "open mole" is generally treated for his/her anxiety by talking to a zoe, who then determines the source of the anxiety. The nursing goal of helping clients to examine sources of their own anxiety was compared to this kind of "talk therapy."

I sought to place emphasis on the treatment of symptoms, rather than on confronting and negating the students' beliefs about **etiology.** Symptoms of mental illness mutually agreed upon included:

(1) withdrawal from social relationships,
(2) singing loudly while pacing the floor, and
(3) wearing dirty and torn clothes.

Each of these symptoms was integrated into discussion of the **symptomatology** of specific mental illnesses. For example, "withdrawal from social relationships" was discussed as part of the symptomatology of schizophrenia and major depressive disorder; "singing loudly while pacing" was discussed as possible symptomatology of **mania;** and "wearing dirty and torn clothes" was discussed as an example of the **unkempt** behavior of a depressed or **psychotic** client.

The belief that the postpartum time is a particularly vulnerable time in which a woman should carry a penknife to ward off spirits was integrated into information about **postpartum depression** and **postpartum psychosis.** Taking someone's clothes away from them while they were in the bush was discussed as a potential safety **precaution** for individuals who were **suicidal.** And, "down-the-line" mental illness was correlated with scientific knowledge that many individuals who suffer from mental illness have a **genetic predisposition** and family history of the illness.

References

Goldberg, J. (1995, Jan. 22). A war without purpose in a country without identity. *The New York Times Magazine, 4,* 36–39.

GPO62-830cc. (1992). The ongoing civil war and crisis in Liberia, 102nd Cong., Ses. 2. (Testimony of Leonard H. Robinson).

Leininger, M. (1970). *Nursing and anthropology: Two worlds to blend.* New York: Wiley.

Leininger, M. (1978). *Transcultural nursing: Concepts, theories, & practices.* New York: Wiley.

Leininger, M. (1985). Transcultural care diversity and universality: A theory of nursing. *Nursing and Health Care, 6,* 209–212.

Leininger, M. (1993). Toward conceptualization of transcultural health care systems: Concepts and a model. *Journal of Transcultural Nursing, 4*(2), 32–40.

Murillo-Rohde, I. (1978). Cultural diversity in curriculum development. In M. Leininger (Ed.), *Transcultural nursing: Concepts, theories, practices* (pp. 451–469). New York: Wiley.

Oyefeso, A. (1994). Attitudes toward the work behaviour of ex-mental patients in Nigeria. *International Journal of Social Psychiatry, 40*(1), 27–34.

Spector, R. (1985). *Cultural diversity in health and illness* (2nd ed.). Norwalk, CT: Appleton-Century-Crofts.

Tripp-Reimer, T., & Lively, S. (1993). Cultural considerations in mental health-psychiatric nursing. In R. Rawlins, S. Williams, & C. Beck (Eds.), *Mental health-psychiatric nursing: A holistic life-cycle approach* (3rd ed., pp. 166–179). St. Louis, MO: Mosby.

Activity: Vocabulary Development

Reading 4.2 contains many mental health and other specialized medical/nursing terms and socio-cultural terms. Add the words you do not know to your dictionary, following the guidelines on page 33. Use a medical English dictionary to look up mental health and other specialized medical/nursing terms and a college-level English dictionary to look up the socio-cultural terms that you do not know. Use 10–15 new words in answering the discussion questions.

Comprehension and Discussion Questions

The questions ask you to locate important information in the reading, as well as think beyond what is stated in the article—for example, by comparing what you have learned about Liberian beliefs about mental illness to your native culture.

1. Look up the word *zoe* in a dictionary. You probably did not find the word. From the information provided in the article, who do you think a *zoe* is? Is there someone like a *zoe* in your native culture? What word is used to refer to a *zoe* in your culture?
2. What are the three main reasons given in Liberia for why someone becomes mentally ill? Are there similar beliefs in your native culture regarding the causes of mental illness? If so, explain how they are similar, as well as how they are different from reasons discussed in the reading.
3. What are the three types of traditional treatments given in Liberia to people who are mentally ill? Are there similar treatments in your native culture? If so, explain how they are similar, as well as different from treatments discussed in the reading.
4. The author wanted to understand traditional Liberian beliefs about mental illness and to integrate that understanding into the way she taught psychiatric nursing to Liberian students. Is the integration of students' cultural beliefs into teaching about psychiatric nursing an important goal? Why or why not?
5. The author compares Liberian beliefs and practices with Western theory and treatment of mental illness. Fill in the chart on page 144 with the corresponding Liberian belief/practice or Western theory/treatment.

Liberian Belief/Practice	Western Theory/Treatment
Spirit's response to wrongdoing	
	Talking about one's feelings with a therapist
Trust in the zoe	
	The therapeutic process
Talking with a zoe, who then determines source of anxiety	
Women who have recently given birth carry a penknife to keep spirits away	
	Safety precaution for individuals who are suicidal
"Down the line" mental illness	

6. The author also compares Liberian and Western understanding of symptoms of mental illness. Fill in the chart with the type of mental illness, as identified in Western theory.

Symptom of mental illness, recognized in both Liberian and Western cultures	Type of mental illness, identified in Western medicine
withdrawal from social relationships	
singing loudly while pacing the floor	
wearing dirty and torn clothes	

Listening to Lectures

Many nursing courses, as well as prerequisite courses, rely heavily on lectures to deliver course content. Your ability to listen and take notes effectively is essential to doing well in those courses.

Your ability to listen effectively to lectures depends on a variety of factors. First, you must have the right attitude. You have to care about listening and make a conscious decision to improve your skills.

Even if the material is difficult or uninteresting, you must see it as a challenge and not tune out. Some of the measures you can take to maximize your listening are:

- Sit up front in the classroom, so you can see and hear clearly.
- Eat before class so you don't get hungry.
- Take a bottle of water with you in case you get thirsty.
- Dress in layers so you can adjust your clothing if you get hot or cold.
- If you hear something you don't agree with, withhold your judgment until you have listened to everything.
- Likewise, do not let preconceived notions about the speaker stop you from listening. Be open to listening to new information and ideas.

Think about the last lecture or long speech you listened to. What happened?

Using the chart, list five reasons (or barriers to) why you have or might have difficulty paying attention to a lecture. Consider such factors as the content of the lecture, location, time, format, delivery style of lecturer, and distractions.

In small groups, discuss strategies for how to overcome each other's barriers to listening. Then, for each of the barriers listed, write a strategy to help you overcome it and stay focused during a lecture. Over the next several weeks, apply these strategies as needed and then write a brief evaluation of each strategy. One has been done for you as an example.

Barriers to Listening	Strategies	Evaluation
1. *My mind sometimes wanders during lectures; I think of things unrelated to the lecture.*	*When my mind begins to wander, I put an exclamation mark in my notes to remind myself to stay focused on the lecture. At the end of the lecture, I count up the number of exclamation marks to see how many times I started to lose focus.*	*I am now more aware of when my mind begins to wander; I am able to stop myself from thinking of other things during lectures.*
2.		
3.		
4.		
5.		

One strategy successful students use to help their listening is to bring a tape recorder to class with them. If you use a tape recorder, you have an accurate record of what was said in class, so you can go back and listen to the lecture or portions of it as often as you need to. This is especially useful when you may have missed a part of the lecture or did not fully understood it. If you and a classmate have different recollections of a point that was made during the lecture, you can use a tape recording to reconcile conflicting notes. If you need to miss class, you can ask a friend to tape record the lecture for you. You can also listen to tapes while you are driving or walking.

Tape-recording lectures, however, does not substitute for effective listening. Students who rely on tape-recording may not pay full attention in class and may take fewer notes because they know they can listen to the tape later. Listening to an entire lecture again on tape is very time-consuming, and you may find that you simply do not have enough time. Also, your tape recorder could malfunction or the recording could be hard to hear. If all you have is a poor recording, you have even less to study from than incomplete notes.

So, while tape-recording lectures can be very helpful, it is best to combine it with active listening and good note-taking skills. Pretend that you are not tape-recording and concentrate as you would without a tape recorder. Use the tape recording selectively after the lecture to review portions of the lecture that are especially important or that you had difficulty understanding, or to clarify or complete your notes.

If you decide to tape-record lectures, ask the instructor first. Sit in the front of the classroom or place the tape recorder as close to the instructor as possible for the best quality recording.

Another effective way to use a tape recorder is to create study tapes. Write a set of study questions, including any Review Questions at the end of assigned units and any questions you have written using learning outcomes or objectives for each unit. (See Unit 1 for further discussion.) Record your study questions, leaving enough time to answer the questions aloud, and then record the answers. Then, when you prepare for a test, test your recall using the study tapes.

Activity: Listening to Lectures and Taking Notes

In this unit, you will practice listening and note-taking skills. First, listen to the lecture on mental health and illness and take notes as best you can. Afterward you will learn about different techniques and strategies that can help you improve your note-taking skills, as well as expand your notes into study guides. After the lecture is over, review your notes as soon as possible. Fill in any missing information by checking with a classmate or the instructor.

Note-Taking Strategies and Skills

It is impossible to write everything that is said in a lecture but, even if you did, you would still have to determine what is important and what is not. Lecturers sometimes go off topic; sometimes they add personal stories or anecdotes; and sometimes they recycle or repeat information. While sometimes these stories and repetitions can help you understand and remember the main points during a lecture, it is not necessary to write them down.

You also do not have time to write your notes out in full form, especially if the instructor is speaking quickly. Fortunately, there are strategies and skills you can learn to be faster and more efficient in your note-taking:

- listening for signal words and phrases
- listening for repetition of phrases and redundancy
- using telegraphic language, symbols, and abbreviations
- listening for stress and intonation

1. Listening for Signal Words and Phrases

Listen for clues that indicate the organizational framework of the lecture, such as words or phrases that signal or mark the introduction, main points in the lecture, and the conclusion.

Words and phrases are also used to introduce points and to indicate the relationship between points.

At the beginning of a lecture, entire sentences may be used to announce the topic, such as:

The topic of today's lecture is . . . .
Today we will look at . . . .
Last class we talked about . . . ; now we will move on to. . . .

Example

In the lecture on mental health and illness, the lecturer begins with: *The topic of today's lecture is mental health and illness.*

Entire sentences are also used to provide additional information about a topic, such as: *There are many reasons for this . . .* or *The symptoms for this illness vary greatly . . . .* Another common technique, often used to introduce a new point, is to refer back to the previous point and then introduce the next point.

Examples

In the lecture on mental health and illness, the lecturer signals the beginning of the first main topic—the condition of mental health—with the following sentence: *First, let's talk about some of the myths and misconceptions that have traditionally surrounded the condition of mental illness.*

Or in moving from one point to the next, the lecturer signals the transition with: *Now that we've looked at mental health, let's look more closely at mental illness.*

Or in restating the main point of a discussion, such as the role of neurotransmitters in the brain: *So we know that there is an influence or incorrect functioning involving neurotransmitters in the brains of individuals suffering from mental disorders.*

Questions can also be used to introduce a main point, explain a main point, or to signal the next main point. Questions that are not meant to be answered by the audience are called **rhetorical questions.** They are helpful in several ways. First, the speaker usually pauses before and after asking them, so you have a little time to catch up with your note-taking. Second, they allow you the opportunity to predict what is coming next. Prediction in listening, as in reading (see page 13 in Unit 1), helps you understand and remember ideas and how they relate to one another.

Examples

In the lecture on mental health and illness, the lecturer introduces temperament as one of the factors influencing mental health. She then asks the question, *Do you know someone who is always upbeat and positive, someone who has a very positive view of life?*

In the discussion of exercise as one of several strategies people use to cope with stress, the lecturer begins with the question, *How does exercise keep us healthy?*

Words and phrases are also used to introduce points or indicate the relationship between points. These words and phrases are called transitions.

order	*first, second, third, next, finally, last*
addition	*in addition, also, furthermore, moreover, besides, and*
contrast	*on the other hand, however, on the contrary, in contrast, otherwise, although*
explanations	*in other words, that is, in fact*
examples	*for example, for instance, to illustrate, such as*
consequence	*as a result, therefore, consequently, thus, for this reason, so*
emphasis	*more important, above all, remember*

Examples

In the lecture on mental health and illness, the lecturer signals at the beginning of the lecture the importance of first addressing stereotypes by stating: ***First,*** *let's talk about some of the myths and misconceptions.*

Or in moving from one point to the next, for example, from family support to life circumstances, the lecturer states: *The* ***last*** *factor that influences mental health is basic life circumstances.*

Or, in providing an example of how technology has improved understanding of mental disorders, the lecturer states: ***For example,*** *in the brain of a depressed person, there is a decrease in the number of certain neurotransmitters.*

Summary statements help to reinforce main points in the lecture. Concluding remarks restate the main points of the lecture, sometimes putting them together in new ways. Transitions, such as *in other words* and *in sum*, are used to introduce summary statements and *in conclusion* and *to summarize* for concluding remarks.

Example

In the lecture on mental health and illness, the lecturer signals the beginning of her concluding remarks with the phrase, ***In conclusion,*** *psychiatric nursing is a very interesting speciality of nursing.*

2. Recognizing Repetition and Redundancy

Main ideas are often stated more than once. You can tell when an idea is important if it is repeated several times, either using the same phrasing or different phrasing.

Example

In the lecture on mental health and nursing, in the discussion of Maslow's Hierarchy of Needs, the lecturer states, *Maslow's Hierarchy represents human* ***needs*** *in the shape of a pyramid. At the bottom of the pyramid are physiological* ***needs,*** *the most basic level of human* ***needs.*** *What are the absolute* ***necessities*** *that we* ***need*** *for life to continue. We* ***have to*** *have oxygen to breathe. Then we* ***need*** *food and water.* The remaining discussion of Maslow's Hierarchy of Needs includes 18 references to needs. By the end of this discussion, it's clear that getting your needs met is an important part of mental health.

3. Using Telegraphic Language

When you take notes, do not write in complete sentences. **Function words,** or words that play a grammatical role in a sentence, are words that can be most easily left out. Examples of function words are: the verb *to be* and other helping verbs, articles, prepositions, and relative pronouns. Words that carry meaning, or **content words,** cannot be left out. Content words are usually nouns, main verbs, adjectives, and adverbs.

The examples are reduced to notes by dropping the function words and writing only the content words. (Note: Telegraphic language is also used in written documentation in nursing.)

Examples

The topic of today's lecture is mental health and illness is reduced to *mental health and illness.*

There are many ways to maintain mental health. One way is through our relationships with other people. Interpersonal relationships, as well as our communication skills with others, are very important. People who are mentally healthy usually have healthy relationships, and they communicate effectively with others. From my practice in nursing, I know that people with mental illness often have difficulties communicating or relating effectively with others. The symptoms of mental illness interfere with the development of healthy interpersonal relationships.

Using telegraphic language, this point is reduced to: *mental health = healthy interpersonal relationships, effective communication skills; mental illness = extreme difficulty communicating effectively.*

Activity: Using Telegraphic Language

Write a telegraphic version for each of the passages that follow.

1. Mental health is a positive state. When we say that someone is mentally healthy, it means that he or she meets certain conditions. According to *Foundations of Psychiatric Mental Health Nursing,* people who are mentally healthy take responsibility for their own actions. They are able to think clearly, use good judgement, and solve problems. Mentally healthy people are aware of their emotional and physical states. They cope effectively with the tensions and stresses of daily living and are able to handle or manage challenges. Mentally healthy people function well in groups, in a family, and in society in general, and they tend to be accepted within those groups. They tend to be satisfied with their lives; they enjoy life and have the ability to find pleasure in living. And, they typically fulfill the capacity for love and work.
   Telegraphic version: ____

   ____

   ____

2. Many factors influence one's mental health. First, we inherit characteristics, or genes, from our parents. Our genetic make-up influences how we cope with life. Our temperament and cognitive abilities are both affected by our genetic make-up and influence how we cope with life. Do you know someone who is always upbeat and positive, someone who has a very positive view of life? That is someone who has a very positive temperament. On the other hand, do you know someone who is negative all the time? The negative person will see a glass that is partially filled with water as half empty, whereas the positive person will see it as half full. Temperament reflects our general outlook on life and the development of our personality. In addition to temperment, our cognitive abilities influence our mental health and again, these are partially determined by our genes. *Cognitive* here means our thinking abilities—processing information, knowing, learning, understanding, and making judgments—all of which influence how mentally healthy we are.
   Telegraphic version: ____

   ____

   ____

3. Besides inherited characteristics, the nurturing received during childhood influences one's mental health. We know from many scientific studies that those first few days, weeks, and years of life are very important. The infant needs to bond with the mother and father; this is very important. We also know that the interactions children have with their family members as they grow and develop are critical in terms of mental health. The influence of support by an extended family can also be a factor. In some cultures the extended family lives together, or they live near each other. In some cases having extended family members around can have a positive influence on a person's mental health, and in times of stress, extended family members can provide support for one another. However, in other cultures, such as the American culture, grandparents and other relatives may live in other states and may not be able to easily provide support. Americans without family members near them may rely on friends or professionals for support instead.
   Telegraphic version: ____

   ____

   ____

4. The last factor that influences mental health is basic life circumstances. Both positive and negative life events can impact or influence our mental health. Witnessing traumatic events, such as tragedies during war or having to leave one's home because of war, as in the case of refugees, can have a negative impact on one's mental health.
   Telegraphic version: ____

   ____

   ____

5. Abraham Maslow was an American psychologist whose most noted contribution to psychology was his "Hierarchy of Needs." This hierarchy provides a good model for understanding the role of needs in the development and maintenance of mental health.
   Telegraphic version: ____

   ____

   ____

4. Using Symbols and Abbreviations

In addition to using telegraphic language in note-taking, symbols and abbreviations can also help you get essential information on paper as quickly as possible.

Symbols

Some symbols that are commonly used in note-taking are:

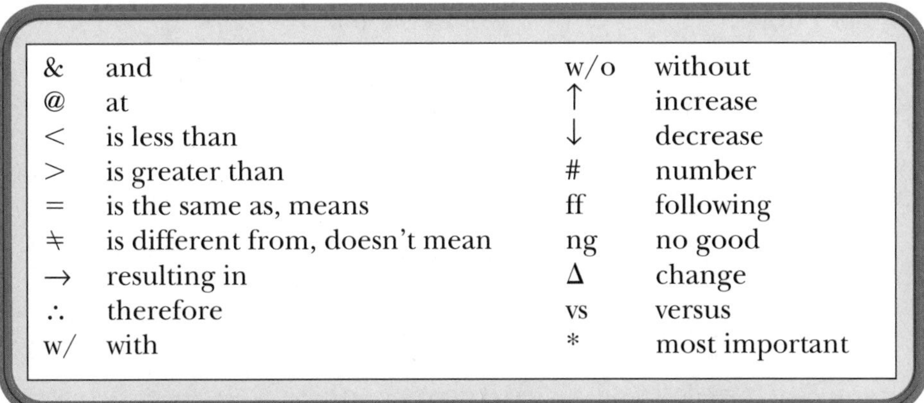

Symbol	Meaning	Symbol	Meaning
&	and	w/o	without
@	at	↑	increase
<	is less than	↓	decrease
>	is greater than	#	number
=	is the same as, means	ff	following
≠	is different from, doesn't mean	ng	no good
→	resulting in	Δ	change
∴	therefore	vs	versus
w/	with	*	most important

You can also create your own symbols, but make sure you record somewhere what each symbol means, in case you forget.

Abbreviations

There are many ways to abbreviate individual words.

Use only the first part of a word.

Examples

medication	*med* (first syllable)
hospital	*hosp* (first syllable and first letter of second syllable)
administration	*admin* (first and second syllable)

Omit vowels and some consonants from the middle of words; retain just enough consonants so you can recognize the word.

Examples

students	*sts*
change	*chng*
years	*yrs*

Use an apostrophe in place of letters in the middle of words.

Examples

international	*int'l*
government	*gov't*

For standard abbreviations, leave off the periods.

Examples

for example (e.g.)	*eg*
compare (c.f.)	*cf*
United States (U.S.)	*US*

Activity: Using Abbreviations

Write an abbreviation for each of the following words or phrases.

Word or Phrase	**Abbreviation**
1. mental health	___________
2. inherited characteristics	___________
3. cognitive abilities	___________
4. childhood nurturing	___________
5. psychologist	___________

5. Recognizing Stress and Intonation

There are several ways in which speakers use their voice to signal important ideas: **volume, pausing,** and **rhythm.** The speaker can raise or lower his or her voice to signal the beginning of an important idea. The speaker can pause before or after stating a main idea to set it apart from the rest of the lecture. Finally, the speaker can use a steady rhythm to introduce a series of important ideas.

Note-Taking Systems

Although there are three common note-taking systems, many people develop their own system over time and it often combines aspects of more than one system. Use whatever system works best for you.

Your instructor may provide you with lecture notes of varying kinds, also referred to as **guided notes.** The most common type is an **outline** or partially completed outline, either formal or informal, of the points covered in the lecture. Another type of guided notes is a handout of **PowerPoint slides.** Next to the content of each slide is space for taking additional notes. An example of guided notes in the form of an outline provided for the mental health lecture is provided.

I. Mental Health: A positive state!
- Self-responsible
- Self-aware
- Thinks clearly, uses good judgment, solves problems
- Copes effectively with daily tension and stress
- Functions well in groups, family, society
- Accepted in groups, family, culture
- Satisfied with and enjoys life
- Fulfills capacity for love and work

    A. Factors influencing mental health
        1. Inherited characteristics
        2. Nurturing during childhood
        3. Support of family and friends
        4. Life circumstances

    B. Maslow's Hierarchy of Needs

    C. Ways to maintain mental health

One common type of note-taking system is outlining, usually an **informal outline** that simply lists main points, with supporting points indented underneath, in contrast to a more formal outline.

Some people learn information more easily when they see it represented in visual form. A **think-link** is a visual map of ideas. When you create a think-link, you use shapes and lines to link main points and supporting points, facts, details, and examples, as shown in Figure 1. Since it would be difficult to create a think-link while listening to a lecture, create an informal outline during class and then afterward, make a think-link from your notes. (Note: A think-link can also be used to brainstorm ideas for a paper.)

Figure 1 Example of a Think-Link—Excerpt from Mental Health and Illness Lecture

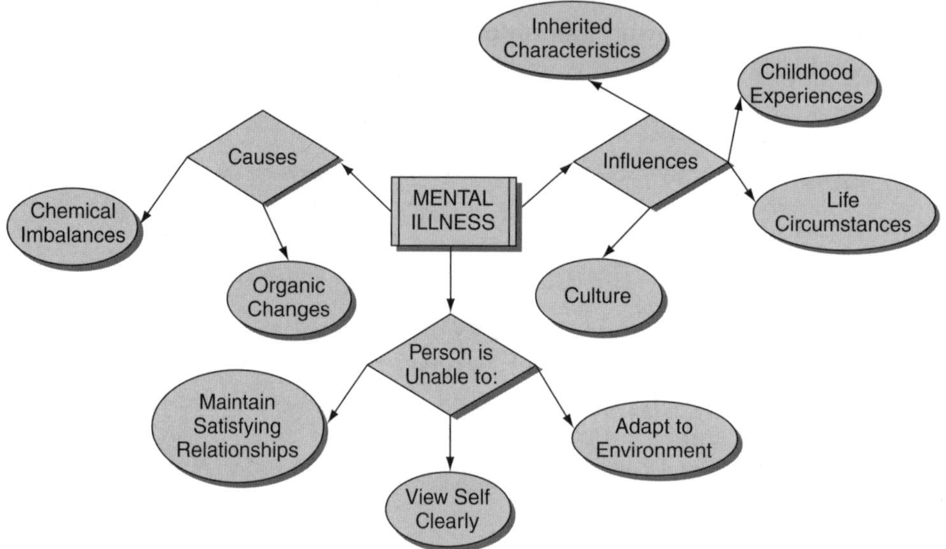

To create a think-link, write the topic of the lecture (or one of the main points) in the middle of a sheet of paper and circle it. Then, draw a line away from the topic, write down the first main idea (or supporting point) at the end of the line, and circle it. Draw lines away from the first main idea; write down specific facts related to that idea and circle each of them. Continue until you have included all the main points and supporting points and important facts, details, or examples in one or more think-links.

In the **Cornell system,** each page is divided into three sections, as shown in Figure 2 on page 157. Section 1, which is the largest section, is located on the right of the page; in this section, you record your notes during the lecture in **informal outline** form. Section 2, to the left of your notes, is the **cue column,** and Section 3, at the bottom of the page, is the **summary area.** The cue column and summary area are filled in after the lecture.

As soon as you can after the lecture, review your notes and fill in the cue column with questions that ask about the main points, or with comments, examples, or visual aids. In the summary area, summarize the notes on the page. Provide an overview of the topic and reinforce the points covered in this part of the lecture. Your summary should answer the questions: *What was the lecture about?* and *What aspects of the topic were covered on this page of notes?*

To use the Cornell system, create the note-taking structure before class or take informal notes during class and then transfer your notes into the Cornell system afterward.

Figure 2 Example of Cornell System—Excerpt from Mental Health and Illness Lecture

May 10, 2008 p.2

Section 2	*Section 1*
What factors influence mental health?	*Factors that influence mental health* *-inherited characteristics (genes from parents)* *-temperament* *-general outlook on life* *-personality*
To what extent do these factors influence mental health or illness?	*-cognitive abilities* *-thinking abilities* *-judgments*
Can these factors cause mental illness?	*-nurturing during childhood* *-early days, weeks, years of life very important* *-infant bonding w/mother and father* *-interaction with family members as child grows and develops very important*
What is the difference between influence and cause?	*-positive influence of extended family*
Is there less mental illness in cultures where people live in extended families or communities?	*-basic life circumstances* *-positive and negative life events* *-witnessing traumatic events; trauma* *-tragedies during war* *-refugees struggle w/this*

Section 3

There are three main factors that can influence a person's mental health: your inherited characteristics, such as temperament and cognitive abilities; the nurturing that you received during childhood, such as the infant bonding with parents, and interactions with other family members growing up; and basic life circumstances, including both positive and negative life events.

Activity: Listening to Lectures and Taking Notes

As you listen again to the lecture on mental health and illness, create an informal outline. After listening to the lecture, compare your notes with a partner or in small groups. Then later, expand your notes, using the Cornell system, or reorganize your notes into think-links.

Apply study strategies to your lecture notes; underline (or highlight) key points, add marginal notes (in note or question format), and anticipate test questions as discussed in Unit 1. The important point is to develop your own system of taking notes and then work with your notes in some way to help commit the information to long-term memory.

Preparing to Be Tested on a Lecture

The quiz on mental health and illness covers the lecture notes and two readings. To prepare for the quiz, anticipate the topics and questions that you think will be asked. Make a list of the main points in both readings. Then write a question for each main point so that by answering the question, you review the relevant information from the reading. Then, review the comprehension and discussion questions. Find the questions that specifically relate to the main points of the readings. Focus on those parts of the readings that answer questions that relate to the main points.

Next, review your lecture notes. What are the topics that were covered in the lecture? For each of the topics listed, write a question. For example, the first topic covered was mental health. Possible questions for that topic are: "What is mental health?" or "How is mental health defined?" or "What are some characteristics of mental health?"

You may need to prioritize what you study from the lecture for the quiz. Some questions to consider as you decide what to focus on in your studying are: What did the instructor spend the most time on in the lecture? What are the most fundamental concepts in the lecture? How does the topic of mental health and illness relate to culture? And, finally, how does the topic of mental health and illness relate to nursing?

Using Note Cards

Take the questions you wrote about the readings and the lecture, and answer them on note cards (with the question on one side and the answer on the other). Then, test yourself. Mix up the note cards so you are not always seeing the information in the same order.

Journal Entry: Reflecting on Mental Health and Illness

Write two or three pages reflecting on what you have learned from the lecture and readings about mental health and illness. Answer the questions.

1. What have you learned in general about mental health and illness from the lecture and readings?
2. How has your understanding and attitude toward mental health and illness changed as a result of the lecture and readings?
3. What difficulties, if any, do you anticipate as a nurse working with mentally ill patients?

UNIT

5

Understanding Quantitative and Qualitative Research in Nursing

The **content-based objectives** include learning about

- Sexuality as a part of nursing practice
- Ways to improve nursing practice related to sexuality
- Issues of sexuality that can interfere with nursing care, such as stereotyping nurses, misunderstanding the use of touch, sexual harassment, and homophobia
- Ways to effectively address issues of sexuality in nursing care

The **skill-based objectives** include

- Research terminology for quantitative and qualitative research
- The organization of a quantitative research article
- Reading and interpreting information in tables
- Interpreting the results of qualitative data analysis

At the end of the unit, you will reflect on your understanding and attitude toward sexuality in nursing and any difficulties you anticipate as a nurse in assessing, treating, and teaching clients about sexuality.

Pre-Reading Activities

Discuss in small groups your answers to these questions. Form groups with classmates who do not have the same cultural background.

1. How is sexuality viewed in your culture?
2. How comfortable are you talking about sexuality?
3. What concerns do you have as a nurse about dealing with sexuality in assessing and treating clients?

Reading Quantitative Research

Reading 5.1 is an example of a quantitative research article. **Quantitative research,** in contrast to qualitative research, uses numbers to understand ideas. Ideas and the relationships between ideas are measured using some kind of objective instrument that gathers numerical data. These data are then analyzed using statistical procedures to determine, for example, their statistical significance and predictive power.

Activity: Understanding the Organization of a Research Article

Preview the reading to locate the main components of a research article. They are listed in the left-hand column.

Components of a Research Article	"Current Nursing Practice Related to Sexuality"
Background to the Study	pp. 167, par. 1–3
Literature Review	________
Purpose of the Study	________
Research Questions	________
Methodology	________
Participants	________
Instrument	________
Procedure	________
Data Analysis	________
Results of the Study	________
Discussion	________
Conclusion	________
Implications	________
Limitations of the Study	________
Recommendations for Future Research	________

Some research articles have headings and subheadings that correspond to each of these components; others do not. Which of these components or categories of information are included in Reading 5.1? Put a check in the blank next to those components that begin with a heading or subheading. If the heading is worded differently in the article than it is in the list, write the wording used in the article. For the categories that are not marked with a heading, write the page and paragraph number where information is provided on that topic. For example, there is no heading in the article for Background to the Study, but background information is provided in the article on page 167, in Paragraphs 1–3 after the abstract.

Make notes in the margin of the article that identify where each component of the research study is located.

Reading and Interpreting Tables

Part of reading about quantitative research involves understanding and interpreting tables. **Tables** display numerical information, usually in columns. **Figures** display information that is usually some combination of numerical and nonnumerical information in another format. (See page 54 for more information about figures.) Tables and figures are often used to support information in an article, so if you are unable to read and correctly interpret the table or figure, you may not understand the information in the reading.

Activity: Reading and Interpreting Tables

Reading 5.1 has four tables. For each table, answer the questions. Unlike when you read and interpreted figures in Unit 2, we have not provided the tables in the activity. Find them in the reading itself.

Table 1: "Number of Respondents by Level of Relevance of Sexuality to Practice Area"

How many columns are included? ______________________________

What does each of the columns refer to? ________________________

In your own words, what is this table showing? ___________________

____

Based on your understanding of Table 1:

1. Is sexuality more important in neurology or mental health? __________
2. Is sexuality more important in intensive care or gerontology? __________
3. Is sexuality more important in rehabilitation or recovery room? _______
4. How many respondents practice in areas where sexuality is least important? __________
5. How many respondents practice in areas where sexuality is moderately important? __________
6. How many respondents practice in areas where sexuality is most impotant? __________

Table 2: "Responses to Questions on Sexuality-Related Nursing Practice"

On the left side of the table, how many questions are listed? __________

Across the top of the table is the label: "Response Categories [n(%)]". Below the label are six categories. What do they refer to? __________

____

In your own words, what is this table showing? __________

____

Based an your understanding of Table 2:

1. What percentage of participants assessed the sexual health of more than 90 percent of their clients during the past year? __________
2. What percentage of participants offered to discuss sexual concerns with more than 50 percent of their clients? __________
3. What percentage of participants provided information to more than 10 percent of their clients? __________
4. What percentage of participants provided counseling to 10 percent or fewer of their clients? __________
5. Note that the response categories are different for the last question listed in the table. What do these response categories refer to? __________

   ____
6. What percentage of participants used a nursing diagnosis for sexuality at least once during the past year? __________

Table 3: "Reported Frequency of Performance of Nursing Activities Related to Patient Sexuality (n = 154)"

On the left side is a list of nursing activities related to patient sexuality.

How many sexuality-related activities are listed? ____________________

On the right side of the table are four different responses. What are they?

____

In your own words, what is this table showing? ____________________

____

Based on your understanding of Table 3:

1. What percentage of participants never assessed the sexual health of their clients during the past year? ____________________
2. What percentage of participants rarely provided teaching about normal sexual development? ____________________
3. What percentage of participants at least occasionally provided teaching about contraception? ____________________
4. What percentage of participants frequently provided teaching about "safe sex"? ____________________
5. Which activity did the most participants participate in at least occasionally? ____________________
6. Which activity did the most participants participate in frequently?

____

Before looking at **Table 4**, read the section in the article on Instrument (see page 169). For each participant in the study, a Practice score was calculated to determine the extent to which nurses addressed sexuality-related concerns in their practice. How was that score calculated? ____________________

____

What was the highest possible Practice score? ____________________

What was the range of Practice scores of participants in the study?

____

Now, read the following excerpt from page 171 about the results of the Practice score and answer the questions that follow.

> Since practice area was coded on relevancy of sexuality in that area, it was hypothesized that the Practice score would differ by practice area. . . . The Practice scores were . . . calculated separately for staff nurses in each practice area. The mean Practice scores for staff nurses working in practice areas coded 1, 2, and 3 were, respectively, 8.2 (n = 25), 9.56 (n = 45), and 16.26 (n = 27). The percentages of nurses in areas coded 1, 2, and 3 with a total Practice score of zero were 36%, 24%, and 4%, *respectively*.

1. What does *respectively* mean? ________________________________
2. What was the Practice score for staff nurses working in a practice area where sexuality was moderately important? __________ most important? __________ least important? ________________________________

   In your own words, what did the researchers hypothesize? ____________

   ____

   What did they find? ____

   Were their findings consistent with their hypothesis? ______________

Table 4: "Regression Analysis of Practice Related to Sexuality on Independent Variables (n=121)"

Table 4 is harder to understand than the other tables. It shows the results of **regression analysis,** a type of statistical analysis that attempts to explain the variation in data. On the left side is a list of variables. How many variables are listed? ____

In the far right column is a list of ***t* values.** The *t* values indicate the relationship between each of the variables listed on the left and practice related to sexuality (measured by the Practice score). You can tell which relationships are **statistically significant** by whether the *t* values have an asterisk next to them. One asterisk indicates that the probability of this relationship occurring by chance is less than 5 percent ($p < 0.05$). Two asterisks indicate that the probability of this relationship occurring by chance is less than 1 percent ($p < 0.01$).

3. One variable has a *p* value of less than 5 percent and four variables have a *p* value of less than 1 percent. What are they? Write them in their order of significance, from most significant to least significant.

   1. ____
   2. ____
   3. ____
   4. ____
   5. ____

In your own words, what do the results of this table indicate?__________

____

____

Together these five variables count for 41 percent of the variance in Practice scores. Look at the **R2** value below the table. That value gives you the percentage of variation due to these five variables. The probability of these relationships occurring by chance is less than 1 in a thousand ($p < 0.001$).

Now, read the following excerpt from page 172 that explains the results of the regression analysis.

The regression indicated that nurses were more likely to include sexuality in their practices if they worked in a hospital in a practice area in which sexuality was particularly relevant, if they believed they had responsibility for discussing sexual concerns, and if they felt knowledgeable and comfortable discussing sexuality. Approximately 41% of the variation in practice related to sexuality was predicted in this regression.

Is your explanation of the results of this table consistent with the explanation in the article? ______________________________

Readings about Sexuality in Nursing

Readings 5.1 and 5.2 discuss some of the ways in which sexuality is part of nursing. As you read these articles, think about similarities and differences between attitudes and practices concerning how sexuality is addressed in the U.S. health care system and in your native culture.

Reading 5.1

Current Nursing Practice Related to Sexuality

Linda K. Matocha, PhD, RN, is an associate professor, and Julie K. Waterhouse, MS, RN, is an assistant professor at the College of Nursing, University of Delaware.

Nurses' practices related to sexuality were examined using the Survey on Sexuality in Nursing Practice (SSNP). The sample consisted of 155 practicing, registered nurses from a variety of practice settings. Twenty percent of subjects indicated they were never involved in any sexuality-related activities and only about 12 percent addressed sexuality with a majority of their clients. Although subjects consistently identified sexuality as a necessary part of nursing practice, few addressed sexual concerns with clients. Weighted least squares analysis of 12 variables revealed that only those variables measuring practice setting and area, nurses' knowledge, responsibility, and comfort were useful predictors of nurses' practice related to sexuality.

The term *sexuality* refers to the "integration of the somatic, emotional, intellectual, and social aspects of sexual being" (World Health Organization, 1975). Nursing practice addressing sexuality is a recognized part of providing holistic client care and may include assessing sexual health, providing anticipatory guidance about sexual development, validating normalcy, educating about sexuality and disease prevention, secondary prevention of disease of the reproductive organs, counseling clients who must adapt to changes in their usual forms of sexual expression, providing intensive therapy for sexual problems, and referring clients to other health care providers (MacElveen-Hoehn, 1985; Poorman, 1988; Waterhouse & Metcalfe, 1991b; Woods, 1984). Sexuality is identified as an important aspect of patient care in nursing and medical literature (Fisher, 1985; Matocha, 1989; Smedley, 1991; Waterhouse & Metcalfe, 1991a; WHO, 1975). However, nurses and physicians often omit counseling about sexual concerns when caring for clients (Calderone, 1980; Ende, Rockwell, & Glasgow, 1984; Metz & Seifert, 1990; Williams, Wilson, Hongladarom, & McDonell, 1986; Young, 1987).

Annon's Permission, Limited Information, Specific Suggestions, and Intensive Therapy model (P–LI–SS–IT) (1974) frequently is utilized to describe levels of sexuality counseling and intervention and provides the conceptual framework for this study (MacElveen-Hoehn, 1985; Rieve, 1989; Smith, 1989; Taylor, Lillis, & LeMone, 1989; Thornton & Dewis, 1989). Permission is the first level of sexuality counseling, and all nurses should be able to function at this level (Annon, 1974; MacElveen-Hoehn, 1985; Rieve, 1989). Permission involves conveying to the client that sexuality is a suitable subject for discussion and providing assurance that concerns or practices are normal. Most nurses can also intervene at the "limited information level" (Rieve, 1989; Thornton & Dewis, 1989). At this level, factual information relevant to the client's concern or problem is given. General sexual concerns, questions, myths, and misconceptions may be addressed.

"Specific suggestions" about sexual concerns and dysfunctions are given at the next level, and "intensive therapy" may be required for severe or long-standing sexual problems (fourth level). Clients needing sexual counseling at level three or four should be referred to an appropriate professional if the nurse providing level one and two counseling lacks the necessary knowledge or skills (MacElveen-Hoehn, 1989; Rieve, 1989).

The needs of several specific groups of patients for sexuality counseling are described in recent literature. Psychiatric clients (Young, 1987), elderly clients (Smedley, 1991), disabled clients (Medhat, Huber, & Medhat, 1990; Rieve, 1989), individuals with cancer (Greenberg, 1987; MacElveen-Hoehn,

1985; Smith, 1989), clients with myocardial infarctions (Baggs & Karch, 1987; McCann, 1989; Tardiff, 1989), poststroke patients (Burgener & Logan, 1989), and clients with multiple sclerosis (Dewis & Thornton, 1989; Thornton & Dewis, 1989) are all represented as requiring nursing intervention in the area of sexuality. Other authors suggest that nurses also should assess sexuality in clients who are apparently healthy or who have minor illnesses (Bachmann, Leiblum, & Grill, 1989; Ende et al., 1984; Metz & Seifert, 1990; Waterhouse & Metcalfe, 1991a).

Several investigators have assessed nurses' opinions about the importance and appropriateness of including sexuality in their nursing care. Overwhelmingly, nurses believed that patient sexuality should be a routine component of nursing care (Shuman & Bohachick, 1987; Smith, 1989; Wilson & Williams, 1988). Despite this general belief, it is often overlooked (Kautz, Dickey, & Stevens, 1990; Shuman & Bohachick, 1987; Wilson & Williams, 1988). Baggs and Karch (1987), Young (1987), and Jenkins (1988) reported that the majority of hospitalized patients received no information about sexuality from nurses or other health care professionals.

Similar practice gaps have been reported in studies of nurses' knowledge and attitudes related to sexuality. Payne (1976), Fisher and Levin (1983), and Webb (1988) reported that nurses lacked knowledge about sexuality and had conservative sexual values. Shuman and Bohachick (1987) found nurses caring for patients with myocardial infarctions to be moderately knowledgeable about sexuality. However, 50% of these nurses reported that they did not feel knowledgeable enough to consistently provide patients with sexual counseling. Similarly, Wilson and Williams (1988) found that oncology nurses frequently cited lack of knowledge as a major reason for not addressing sexuality concerns.

Lief and Payne (1975) reported a significant positive correlation between sexual knowledge and attitudes and nurses' behavior in patient care situations involving sexuality. Similarly, Wilson and Williams (1988) found a significant correlation between oncology nurses' sexual attitudes and self-reported behaviors addressing sexuality with clients. Other investigators have shown that more education in sexuality generally results in higher knowledge levels in the area of sexuality, but increases have been very modest (Aja & Self, 1986; Katzman & Katzman, 1987; Roy, 1983; Schnarch & Jones, 1981; Whatley, 1986; Woods & Mandetta, 1975). Effects of education on attitudes and actual practice are even less clear.

Previous investigators have examined nursing practice related to sexuality only in specific practice areas or settings (Kautz et al., 1990; Shuman & Bohachick, 1987; Wilson & Williams, 1988). The primary purpose of this pilot study was to identify the extent to which nurses in a wide variety of practice settings discussed sexual concerns with their patients. A second purpose was to identify the influences of practice area, practice position, education, values, opinions, and demographics on sexuality-related nursing practice.

Method

Sample

The **population** sampled included practicing, registered nurses in a South-Atlantic state. A systematic probability sample of 500 potential subjects was obtained by selecting every 17th nurse from a list of currently licensed registered nurses supplied by the state's Board of Nursing. One hundred fifty-five nurses (31%) responded to a questionnaire assessing their practice related to sexuality.

The typical subject was female (98%), Caucasian (93%), married (73%), between 30 and 50 years of age (72%), had a diploma or baccalaureate education (68%), worked in a hospital setting (52%), and held a position of staff nurse (63%). The majority (73%) had had no continuing education on sexuality in nursing practice, and most (80%) considered their personal values about sexuality to be average to much less conservative than average. The sample characteristics for gender, age, race, and marital status did not differ significantly from Groff's (1987) descriptive survey of nurses in the state.

Instrument

The Survey on Sexuality in Nursing Practice (SSNP) was developed for use in this pilot study and was based conceptually on Annon's model with specific **variables** derived from appropriate nursing practices found in reviewing the literature. Only those practices at the "permission" and "limited information" levels of Annon's model were included because all nurses should be expected to intervene at these levels. In addition, items measuring **demographic data,** perceived comfort, knowledge, and responsibility toward sexuality in nursing practice, personal values related to sexuality, and continuing education on sexuality were measured. Questions were designed for subjects with at least a grade 12 reading level. The SSNP was a self-report questionnaire composed of 36 multiple choice, 5 short answer, and 1 open-ended question, producing **nominal** and **ordinal** level **data.**

Practice in sexuality was measured as the percentage of clients with whom the nurse had addressed sexuality in the past year, and the frequency with which she/he had performed various sexuality-related nursing activities. The responses to the frequency questions were scored 0= never to 3=frequently, and these frequency scores were totaled to yield an overall practice related to sexuality score (PRACTICE) (range from 0 to 30). Three items tested perceived knowledge level related to sexuality, opinion about nurses' responsibility to include sexuality in practice, and nurses' comfort level when discussing sexual concerns. Item responses were measured on scales with five response levels (1=never/not at all to 5=extremely/always). There was one short answer question regarding subjects' participation in continuing education and staff development programs related to sexuality (1=none to 3=more than 8 hr). Another question asked subjects to rate their belief about their personal values about sexuality on a 5-point scale ranging from much more conservative than most peoples' (1) to much less conservative (5).

The practice area variable was coded 1, 2, or 3 based on theoretical relevance of practice in sexuality for that area as documented in literature. Practice areas coded 1 represented areas in which sexuality would less frequently be an important focus, while practice areas coded 3 were those in which the literature indicated sexuality should be a frequent and essential focus of nursing care. For example, gynecology, postpartum and psych-mental health were coded 3 (Jenkins, 1988; Krueger et al., 1979; Nurses' Association of the American College of Obstetrics and Gynecologists, 1981; Young, 1987). Gerontology, pediatrics, and oncology were coded 2 (American Nurses' Association & Oncology Nursing Society, 1987; Talashek, Tichy, & Epping, 1990; Whaley & Wong, 1991). Operating room and nursery were coded 1 (Bobak, Jensen, & Zalar, 1989; Gruendemann & Meeker, 1987). Numbers of nurses and practice areas included in each level are indicated in Table 1. Demographic data included age (20–29=1 to 60–69=5), race (*Caucasian*=1 and *other*=0), marital status (*married*=1 and *other*=0), place of employment (*hospital*=1 and *other*=0), and position (*staff nurse*=1 and *other*=0).

Content validity of the SSNP was established by four expert reviewers: one doctorally-prepared and two masters-prepared nurses with expertise in sexuality and a variety of clinical areas, and a doctorally-prepared expert in measurement and statistics. The results of the reviews indicated that the survey was appropriate and adequately measured nursing practice related to issues in sexuality. The questions were pretested for clarity on 81 junior and senior nursing students. An item analysis was conducted which included item discriminations and overall alpha level. Items were refined or eliminated based on reviewers' comments and item analysis results. The **Cronbach alpha level** of the revised questionnaire was .93. **Test-retest reliability** was not measured in this initial phase of instrument development.

Results

Responses to questions on the percentage of clients with whom the nurse's practice included sexuality are presented in Table 2. Thirty-four percent of the subjects had not assessed sexual health in

Table 1 Number of Respondents by Level of Relevance of Sexuality to Practice Area

Level of Relevance	Practice Area	n
Least important	Anesthesiology	1
(code = 1)	Emergency room	8
	Intensive care	17
	Nursery	3
	Operating room	1
	Quality assurance	3
	Recovery room	2
	Other	8
Moderately	Gerontology	14
important	Labor/delivery	4
(code = 2)	Medical	18
	Neurology	3
	Oncology	9
	Orthopedics	5
	Pediatrics	8
	Surgical	6
	Other	
Most important	Community health	15
(code = 3)	Gynecology	6
	HIV	2
	Postpartum	2
	Mental health	9
	Rehabilitation	5
	Other	3

any client during the past year, and another 44% had assessed sexual health in 10% or fewer of their clients. Similarly, 75% offered to discuss sexual concerns with 10% or fewer of their clients, and 71% provided sexuality information to 10% or fewer of their clients. Ninety-three percent initiated referrals related to sexuality for 10% or fewer of their clients in the past year. Only 5% indicated that nursing diagnoses were not used in their facility, but 72% indicated that they had never used the nursing diagnoses "Sexual Dysfunction" or "Altered Sexuality Patterns" during the past year. Only 31% of subjects believed they were very or extremely knowledgeable about sexuality; 59% of the sub-

Table 2 Responses to Questions on Sexuality-Related Nursing Practice

	Response Categories [n(%)]					
Questions	0%	<2%	2–10%	11–50%	51–90%	>90%
Assessed sexual health?	52(34.2)	34(34.2)	30(19.7)	19(12.5)	9(5.9)	8(5.3)
Offered to discuss sexual concerns?	41(26.8)	41(26.8)	33(21.6)	19(12.4)	14(9.2)	5(3.3)
Provided information?	47(30.4)	34(22.2)	28(18.3)	23(15.0)	11(7.2)	10(6.5)
Provided counseling?	80(52.6)	44(28.9)	17(11.2)	8(5.3)	1(0.7)	2(1.3)
	0 times	<5 times	6–10 times	11–25 times	>25 times	Not used
Used nursing diagnosis for sexuality?	110(71.9)	23(15.0)	7(4.6)	2(1.3)	3(2.0)	8(5.2)

jects thought that nurses usually or always had a responsibility to discuss sexual concerns with clients, and 69% reported that they were usually or always comfortable discussing sexual concerns.

The frequencies with which subjects were involved in various nursing practices that relate to sexuality are presented in Table 3. For each of the 10 sexuality-related activities, between 26% and 47% of subjects had never been involved in the activity, and between 44% and 87% rarely or never had been involved in the activity. Answering clients' questions about sexuality and listening to clients' concerns about sexuality were the activities engaged in most frequently. Fifty-six percent of subjects answered their clients' sexuality questions occasionally or frequently, but 44% of subjects rarely or never answered questions. Similarly, 52% listened to concerns about sexuality occasionally or frequently, but 48% rarely or never listened to these concerns. The activities least often engaged in were teaching testicular self-exam and teaching normal sexual development.

Total PRACTICE scores for the subjects ranged from 0 to 28 out of the potential 30 (M = 11.48, SD = 8.65). Twenty percent of subjects indicated they were never involved in any of the 10 activities. Total scores for an additional 24% of subjects fell between 0 and 10, indicating they rarely or never performed most activities. Only 16% of subjects scored above 20 on the composite score, indicating that they performed most activities occasionally to frequently.

Since practice area was coded on relevancy of sexuality in that area, it was **hypothesized** that the PRACTICE score would differ by practice area. In addition, it was thought that these scores might also depend on practice position, since nurses working in positions such as nurse manager, staff development, and faculty would have much less direct client contact than would staff nurses. The PRACTICE scores were, therefore, calculated separately for staff nurses in each practice area. The mean PRACTICE scores for staff nurses working in practice areas coded 1, 2 and 3 were, respectively, 8.2 (n = 25), 9.56 (n = 45), and 16.26 (n = 27). The percentages of nurses in areas coded 1, 2, and 3 with a total PRACTICE score of zero were 36%, 24%, and 4%, respectively.

Ordinary least squares regression was used to explore the influence of 12 independent variables on practices related to sexuality. Although **dichotomous variables** are sometimes excluded from **regression analyses,** it was appropriate and statistically valid in this study to include race, marital status, practice place, and practice position as dummy variables (Tabachnick & Fidell, 1989; Tatsuoka, 1988). Practice area, place of employment, perceived knowledge level, perceived responsibility, and comfort were **significant predictors** of practices in sexuality (Table 4). To correct for

Table 3 Reported Frequency of Performance of Nursing Activities Related to Patient Sexuality (n = 154)

	Responses [n (%)]			
Activities	Never	Rarely	Occasionally	Frequently
Assessment of sexual health	59(38.3)	38(24.7)	37(24.0)	20(13.0)
Teaching about normal sexual development	62(40.3)	54(35.1)	22(14.3)	16(10.4)
Teaching about sexually transmitted diseases	57(37.0)	25(16.2)	41(26.6)	31(20.1)
Teaching breast self-examination	63(40.9)	37(24.0)	31(20.1)	23(14.9)
Teaching testicular self-examination	72(46.8)	63(40.9)	12 (7.8)	7 (4.5)
Teaching about contraception	61(39.6)	38(24.7)	31(20.1)	24(15.6)
Teaching about "safe sex"	60(39.0)	33(21.4)	33(21.4)	28(18.2)
Teaching modification in sexual practice	62(40.3)	30(19.5)	43(27.9)	19(12.3)
Answering questions about sexuality	41(26.6)	27(17.5)	60(39.0)	26(16.9)
Listening to concerns about sexuality	40(26.0)	34(22.1)	53(34.4)	27(17.5)

heteroscedasticity in the data, a weighted least squares (WLS) approach was used to calculate correct **t values.** The WLS approach yielded the same five predictors.

The regression indicated that nurses were more likely to include sexuality in their practices if they worked in a hospital in a practice area in which sexuality was particularly relevant, if they believed they had responsibility for discussing sexual concerns, and if they felt knowledgeable and comfortable discussing sexuality. Approximately 41% of the variation in practice related to sexuality was predicted in this regression.

Discussion

According to Annon's (1974) model, all practicing nurses should be able to give "permission" and provide "limited information" to their clients regarding sexuality. The results of this study suggest that many nurses are not meeting these responsibilities for client care in the area of sexuality. Results confirm previous outcomes showing that nursing practice related to sexuality is inadequate based on existing nursing standards (American Nurses' Association, 1980). At least one third of these nurses never assessed sexual health, discussed sexuality with clients, or taught about sexuality. Even fewer made referrals or used nursing diagnoses for sexuality. Further, a very small proportion of subjects routinely addressed sexuality with all or a majority of their clients.

The scores on the combined PRACTICE variable gave evidence that current sexuality-related nursing care is insufficient. There was no expectation that all nurses should be involved in all of the 10 sexuality-related activities. For example, higher average PRACTICE scores for staff nurses in

Table 4 Regression Analysis of Practice Related to Sexuality on Independent Variables (n = 121)

Variable	Beta	Std. Beta	*SE* Beta	T_{wls}
Age	0.096	0.011	0.810	0.10
Race	-2.001	-0.588	2.698	-1.00
Marital status	0.743	0.391	1.482	0.51
Practice place	4.235	0.250	1.567	2.73**
Position	-1.623	-0.093	1.448	-1.20
Practice area	3.424	0.314	0.997	3.30**
Education	-0.544	-0.063	0.693	-0.87
Continuing education	1.967	0.160	1.150	1.87
Personal values	0.268	0.029	0.765	0.36
Knowledge	3.171	0.253	1.048	3.50**
Responsibility	1.711	0.180	0.742	2.32*
Comfort	2.279	0.222	0.866	2.80**

Note. Multiple R = .637, R^2 = .406, $F_{(12, 108)}$ = 6.12, and $p < 0.001$.
Note. WLS = Weighted Least Squares.
**$p < 0.01$. *$p < 0.05$.

highly relevant practice areas indicated that nurses were addressing sexuality more often in these areas. However, sexuality-related practice was infrequent in all practice areas. Even more troublesome was the fact that 36% of staff nurses in areas coded least relevant and 24% of staff nurses in areas coded moderately relevant were *never* involved in any nursing activities related to sexuality.

The only activities related to sexuality which were performed occasionally to frequently by a majority of nurses were "listening to clients' concerns" and "answering questions about sexuality." These are both *client-initiated* activities, rather than interventions initiated by nurses. This parallels findings by Wilson and Williams (1988) and Smith (1989) showing that nurses wait for clients to initiate discussions about sexuality.

Subjects' positive perceptions of nurses' responsibility to discuss sexuality with clients provided a sharp contrast to the low practice scores. These nurses clearly believed that they had a responsibility to discuss sexuality with clients, supporting Shuman and Bohachick's (1987) results. The finding that the subjects were comfortable discussing sexuality matches Williams et al.'s (1986) finding that 67% of nurses were comfortable talking with clients about sexuality. The majority of nurses in this study believed that they were only somewhat knowledgeable about sexuality, paralleling earlier results (Shuman & Bohachick, 1987; Wilson & Williams, 1988). The fact that the percentage of nurses who usually or always felt comfortable discussing sexuality exceeded the percentage who felt very or extremely knowledgeable by 38 percent is surprising. Generally, knowledge about a particular nursing intervention should be a prerequisite for feeling comfortable with the procedure. Perhaps the subjects really meant that they would feel comfortable discussing sexuality if and when they had the required knowledge.

It was expected that age, marital status, practice position, basic education, continuing education, and personal values might each influence nurses' practice related to sexuality; however, none of these variables was a significant predictor. The fact that practice area significantly predicted PRACTICE was anticipated because practice areas were coded based on the relevance of practice in sexuality for that area. It is difficult to explain why place of employment significantly predicted practice related to sexuality, and particularly why hospital nurses were more likely to address sexuality than nurses employed in other settings. Sexuality is certainly an important topic in school nursing, home health and community nursing, physicians' offices, occupational health, and many other nonhospital settings. The fact that perceived knowledge and comfort were more important predictors than was perceived responsibility is intriguing. Apparently many nurses recognized that they have a responsibility to discuss sexuality, but were only likely to do so if they felt knowledgeable and comfortable.

Overall, results of this study indicate that many nurses rarely include sexuality discussions in their practices and that only practice area and place and nurses' perceived knowledge, comfort, and responsibility are useful predictors of the extent of nurses' practice related to sexuality. The study sample was adequate in size (Tabachnick & Fidell, 1989) and appeared to be representative of the total population of nurses in the state. However, the sample **response rate** was only 31%, and subjects volunteered to participate. This may have introduced a selection bias, because individuals who agree to complete a questionnaire on sexuality in nursing practice are likely to have more interest in the subject than individuals who do not volunteer (Fowler, 1988). This implies that the 345 nurses contacted who did not return the SSNP may have been even less likely to include sexuality in their practices than those who completed the survey. Other potential limitations of this study included use of a new instrument for which minimal **reliability** and **validity** were established, and the fact that only 41% of the variance in practice related to sexuality was accounted for by the study variables. This implies that at least one, and possibly several important variables were omitted from the study. Another limitation was the measurement of perceived knowledge, comfort, responsibility, and values with only one item each. Measurement of these variables with several items would have increased the reliability of the measurements.

This study was intended as a **pilot** for more extensive research, and results are certainly not conclusive. Nevertheless, it raises numerous questions that should stimulate further study. Why are hospital nurses more likely to include sexuality in their practices than nurses in other settings? Does continuing education on sexuality really change nursing practice related to sexuality? What factors influence nurses' attitudes toward sexuality-related practice, and how, specifically, do these attitudes influence practice? Hopefully, answers to some of these questions will allow nursing to provide higher quality of care for all clients. It is of vital importance that nurses address the sexual concerns of all clients, particularly today, as incidences of HIV infection and teenage pregnancy reach critical levels. Nurses who do not address sexuality when appropriate fail to meet their professional responsibilities in this essential area. The findings of this study provide evidence that there is considerable room for improvement in nurses' current practice related to sexuality.

References

Aja, A., & Self, D. (1986). Alternate methods of changing nursing home staff attitudes toward sexual behavior of the aged. *Journal of Sex Education and Therapy, 12*, 37–41.

American Nurses' Association. (1980). *Nursing: A social policy statement.* Kansas City, MO: Author.

American Nurses' Association and Oncology Nursing Society. (1987). *Standards of oncology nursing practice.* Kansas City, MO: Authors.

Annon, J. S. (1974). *The behavioral treatment of sexual problems.* Honolulu, HI: Enabling Systems.

Bachmann, G. A., Leiblum, S. R., & Grill, J. (1989). Brief sexual inquiry in gynecologic practice. *Obstetrics and Gynecology, 73*, 425–427.

Baggs, J. G., & Karch, A. M. (1987). Sexual counseling of women with coronary heart disease. *Heart & Lung, 16*, 154–159.

Bobak, I. M., Jensen, M. D., & Zalar, M. K. (1989). *Maternity and gynecologic care.* Baltimore, MD: Mosby.

Burgener, S., & Logan, G. (1989). Sexuality concerns of the poststroke patient. *Rehabilitation Nursing, 14*, 178–181, 195.

Calderone, M. S. (1980). Doctor, will it leave a scar? *Frontiers of Radiation Therapy Oncology, 14*, 130–133.

Dewis, M. W., & Thornton, N. G. (1989). Sexual dysfunction in multiple sclerosis. *Journal of Neuroscience Nursing, 21*, 175–179.

Ende, M. D., Rockwell, S., & Glasgow, M. (1984). The sexual history in general medicine practice. *Archives of Internal Medicine, 144*, 558–561.

Fisher, S. G. (1985). The sexual knowledge and attitudes of oncology nurses: Implications for nursing education. *Seminars in Oncology Nursing, 1*, 63–68.

Fisher, S., & Levin, D. (1983). The sexual knowledge and attitudes of professional nurses caring for oncology patients. *Cancer Nursing, 6*, 55–62.

Fowler, F. J., Jr. (1988). *Survey research methods.* Newbury Park, CA: Sage.

Greenberg, D. B. (1987). The measurement of sexual dysfunction in cancer patients. *Cancer, 53*, 2281–2285.

Groff, L. (1987). *1987 survey of RNs in Delaware* (Internship Report). Dover, DE: Delaware Nurses' Association.

Gruendemann, B. J., & Meeker, M. H. (1987). *Care of the patient in surgery.* Washingon, DC: Mosby.

Jenkins, B. (1988). Patient's reports of sexual changes after treatment for gynecological cancer. *Oncology Nursing Forum, 5*, 349–354.

Katzman, E. M., & Katzman, L. S. (1987). Outcomes of sexuality course in nursing education. *Journal of Sex Education and Therapy, 13*, 33–36.

Kautz, D. D., Dickey, D. A., & Stevens, M. N. (1990). Using research to identify why nurses do not meet established sexuality nursing care standards. *Journal of Nursing Quality Assurance, 4*(3), 69–78.

Krueger, J. C., Hassell, J., Goggins, B. B., Ishimatso, T., Pablico, M. R., & Tuttle, E. J. (1979). Relationship between nurse counseling and sexual adjustment after hysterectomy. *Nursing Research, 28*, 145–150.

Lief, H. I., & Payne, T. (1975). Sexuality-knowledge and attitudes. *American Journal of Nursing, 75*, 2026–2029.

MacElveen-Hoehn, P. (1985). Sexual assessment and counseling. *Seminars in Oncology Nursing, 1*, 69–75.

Matocha, L.K. (1989). The effects of AIDS of family member(s) responsible for care: A qualitative study. *Dissertation Abstracts International* (University Microfilms No. 90–19, 300).

McCann, M. E. (1989). Sexual healing after heart attack. *American Journal of Nursing, 89*, 1132–1138.

Medhat, A., Huber, P. M., & Medhat, M. (1990). Factors that influence the level of activity in persons with lower extremity amputation. *Rehabilitation Nursing, 15*, 13–18.

Metz, M. E., & Seifert, M. H. (1990). Men's expectations of physicians in sexual health concerns. *Journal of Sex and Marital Therapy, 16,* 79–88.

Nurses' Association of the American College of Obstetricians and Gynecologists (NAACOG). (1981). *Standards for obstetric, gynecologic, and neonatal nursing.* Washington, DC: Author.

Payne, T. (1976). Sexuality of nurses: Correlations of knowledge, attitudes, and behavior. *Nursing Research, 25,* 286–292.

Poorman, S. G. (1988). *Human sexuality and the nursing process.* Norwalk, CT: Appleton & Lange.

Rieve, J. E (1989). Sexuality and the adult with acquired physical disability. *Nursing Clinics of North America, 24,* 265–276.

Roy, J. H. (1983). A study of knowledge and attitudes of selected nursing students toward human sexuality. *Issues in Health Care of Women, 4,* 127–137.

Schnarch, D. M., & Jones, K. (1981). Efficacy of sex education courses in medical school. *Journal of Sex and Marital Therapy, 7,* 307–317.

Shuman, N. A., & Bohachick, P. (1987). Nurses' attitudes towards sexual counseling. *Dimensions of Critical Care Nursing, 6,* 75–80.

Smedley, G. (1991). Addressing sexuality in the elderly. *Rehabilitation Nursing, 16,* 9–11.

Smith, D. B. (1989). Sexual rehabilitation of the cancer patient. *Cancer Nursing, 12,* 10–15.

Tabachnick, B. G., & Fidell, L. S. (1989). *Using multivariate statistics.* New York: Harper & Row.

Talashek, M. L., Tichy, A. M., & Epping, H. (1990). Sexually transmitted diseases in the elderly: Issues and recommendations. *Journal of Gerontological Nursing, 16,* 33–40.

Tardiff, G. S. (1989). Sexual activity after a myocardial infarction. *Archives of Physical Medicine and Rehabilitation, 70,* 763–766.

Tatsuoka, M. M. (1988). *Multivariate analysis: Techniques for educational and psychological research.* New York: Macmillan.

Taylor, C., Lillis, C., & LeMone, P. (1989). *Fundamentals of nursing: The art and science of nursing care.* Philadelphia: J.B. Lippincott.

Thornton, N. G., & Dewis, M. (1989). Multiple sclerosis and female sexuality. *Canadian Nurse, 85*(4), 16–18.

Waterhouse, J. K., & Metcalfe, M. C. (1991a). Altered sexuality patterns. In L.J. Carpenito, *Nursing diagnosis: Application to clinical practice.* Philadelphia: Lippincott.

———. (1991b). Attitudes toward nurses discussing sexual concerns with patients. *Journal of Advanced Nursing, 6,* 1048–1054.

Webb, D. (1988). A study of nurses' knowledge and attitudes about sexuality in health care. *International Journal of Nursing Studies, 25,* 235–244.

Whaley, L. F., & Wong, D. L. (1991). *Nursing care of infants and children* (4th ed.). Washington, DC: Mosby.

Whatley, M. H. (1986). Integrating sexuality issues into the nursing curriculum. *Journal of Sex Education and Therapy, 12,* 23–26.

Williams, H. A., Wilson, M. E., Hongladarom, G., & McDonell, M. (1986). Nurses' attitudes towards sexuality in cancer patients. *Oncology Nursing Forum, 13*(2), 39–43.

Wilson, M. E., & Williams, H. A. (1988). Oncology nurses' attitudes and behaviors related to sexuality of patients with cancer. *Oncology Nursing Forum, 15,* 49–52.

Woods, N. F. (1984). *Human sexuality in health and illness.* St. Louis, MO: Mosby.

Woods, N. F., & Mandetta, A. F. (1975). Changes in students' knowledge and attitudes following a course in human sexuality: Report of a pilot study. *Nursing Research, 4,* 10–15.

World Health Organization. (1975). *Education and treatment in human sexuality: The training of health professionals.* Technical Report Series (No. 572). Geneva: WHO.

Young, E. W. (1987). Sexual needs of psychiatric clients. *Journal of Psychosocial Nursing, 25,* 30–32.

Research Terminology

Reading 5.1 contains many words about quantitative research design and statistical procedures.

Activity: Understanding Research Terminology

Match each word about research design and statistical procedures with its definition.

Research Design

a. pilot
b. hypothesize
c. instrument
d. content validity
e. variables
f. demographic data
g. population
h. validity
i. sample
j. response rate
k. reliability

1. ____________________:
The extent to which an instrument measures what it claims to measure, by including a representative sampling of items.
2. ____________________:
To suggest a possible explanation that has not yet been proven to be true.
3. ____________________:
The percentage of persons who were initially contacted to participate in a study and that actually participated.
4. ____________________:
The extent to which the results of a test or measure are consistent or stable.
5. ____________________:
The extent to which a test or instrument measures what it claims to be measuring.
6. ____________________:
A small study that is conducted to test an instrument for its validity and reliability and/or to determine the feasibility of a larger study.
7. ____________________:
A subgroup taken from the group that is of interest in a study, usually randomly selected in a quantitative study.
8. ____________________:
The entire group that is of interest in a study.
9. ____________________:
The means by which data is collected in a study.
10. ____________________:
Human characteristics or abilities that differ over time or among individuals.
11. ____________________:
Characteristics about the participants in a study, such as age, gender, occupation, etc.

Statistical Procedures

a. dichotomous variables
b. ordinal data
c. significant predictors
d. nominal data
e. regression analysis
f. test-retest reliability
g. Cronbach alpha level
h. *t* values

1. ____________________:
   Data that identify groups or categories of people, such as male/female or nationality.
2. ____________________:
   Data that are used to order or rank information, such as on a scale of 1 to 5, with 1 representing the best and 5 the worst.
3. ____________________:
   The most common way of testing the reliability of an instrument is by dividing the scores into two halves, usually by even and odd numbers, and calculating the relationship between the scores on the two subtests, resulting in a correlation coefficient.
4. ____________________:
   One way of testing the reliability of an instrument is by administering it twice to one group of subjects on two different occasions and calculating the relationship between the two sets of scores.
5. ____________________:
   A type of nominal variable in which there are only two options, such as male/female.
6. ____________________:
   A statistical procedure used to estimate a person's performance on one variable from the performance on one or more other variables.
7. ____________________:
   Variables that have been shown to affect a person's performance on another variable at a statistically significant level.
8. ____________________:
   The results of a statistical procedure, called the *t*-test, that is used to compare the means of two groups on a measure.

Comprehension and Discussion Questions

The questions ask you to locate important information in the article, as well as analyze carefully and think critically about information in the reading.

1. What are some ways in which sexuality is part of the holistic care of clients?
2. What is the PLISSIT model and what is it used for?
3. What do each of the levels in the PLISSIT model stand for (P, LI, SS, IT)? Which two levels should all nurses be competent in providing?
4. What instrument used in this study is based on the PLISSIT model?
5. What do "listening to clients' concerns" and "answering [clients'] questions about sexuality" have in common? Why is this a source of concern for the researchers?
6. On page 173, the authors state: "The fact that the percentage of nurses who usually or always felt comfortable discussing sexuality exceeded the percentage who felt very or extremely knowledgeable by 38% is surprising." Why is this finding surprising, according to the authors? Do you find it surprising? Why or why not?
7. The authors expected a number of variables to influence nurses' practice related to sexuality. Which variables predicted nurses' practice related to sexuality? Which variables did not? (*Hint:* See Table 4.)
8. What is a **selection bias**? Was there a selection bias in the study's respondents? If so, what does it suggest for the findings of this study? Does the bias strengthen or weaken the researchers' findings? Explain your answer.
9. In this study, "place of practice" was a significant predictor of nurses' practice related to patient sexuality, specifically hospital nurses were more likely to include sexuality in their practice than nurses in non-hospital settings, such as school nursing, home health and community nursing, physicians' offices, and occupational health. Why do you think hospital nurses are more likely than nurses in other settings to include sexuality in their practice?
10. Why is it especially important in today's world for nurses to address the sexual concerns of all clients? What are some other reasons, besides those given in the reading?

Reading Qualitative Research

Qualitative research is much different from quantitative research because there are no numbers to crunch and, therefore, no statistical procedures to be carried out. Data are often collected through interviews with participants, as in "Nurses' Perceptions of Sexuality Relating to Patient Care," observation, and/or document analysis. There are no specific hypotheses to be proved or disproved in qualitative research, but rather broad conceptual issues to be explored with the participants. Likewise, there are no predetermined categories of analysis; rather, those categories emerge from analysis of the data for reoccurring themes. Data are also collected in the natural environment in which the focus of interest occurs. Usually there are far fewer participants in qualitative research than in quantitative research studies, and they are not randomly selected. This means researchers cannot generalize their data to the larger group or population represented by participants, but the data that are collected are much richer and potentially more meaningful than quantitative data, which by their very nature are limited to what is measurable in discrete categories.

Activity: Understanding the Results of Qualitative Data Analysis

In qualitative research, the data can be overwhelming, so it is especially important to understand how the data have been analyzed and reported. In Reading 5.2, only headings, not subheadings, have been used in presenting and discussing the results of the study. Skim the section Description and Discussion of Findings. Complete the outline, adding subheadings for each of the broad conceptual themes of *talking, stereotyping,* and *coping.* A few items have been done for you. Note that in an outline, I, II, and III represent the most general level of information and i. and ii. the most specific level. Then, write notes in the margin of the text, identifying the location of information associated with each subheading.

I. Talking

A. Initiation

1. *Patient should initiate discussion on sexuality*

B. Upbringing

1. ______________________________

2. *Sexuality as taboo subject*

C. ______________________________

1. Prevents nurses from establishing close relationships with patients

D. Logistics

1. ______________________________

2. Heavy workload

E. ______________________________

F. Priority of care

1. Sexuality not a priority, especially in acute surgical settings

II. Stereotyping

A. Stereotypes of nurses

1. ______________________________

2. Role of the media in creating negative images

3. ______________________________

a. White

b. ______________________________

B. Sexual harassment

1. Female nurse as sex object

2. ______________________________

a. Taboo body parts exposed

b. ______________________________

3. Use of touch

a. ______________________________

b. Touch is routine for nurses

4. ______________________________

C. Homosexual patients

1. ______________________________

2. Nursing care of homosexual patients is inadequate

III. Coping

A. ______________________________

1. With intimate, invasive procedures
2. ______________________________
   a. Nurses touch or come too close to patients
   b. ______________________________
3. Events given inappropriate sexual connotations
   a. Caring for homosexual patients
   b. ______________________________

B. Coping strategies

1. Avoidance of patients
2. ______________________________
   a. "Coercive power"—way nurses can assert power
   b. ______________________________
      i. Detract from standard of care
      ii. Remain in place unless patient behaves in acceptable manner
3. ______________________________
   a. Claims event that caused embarrassment is routine
   b. ______________________________
4. ______________________________
   a. At expense of patients
   b. Shared with patients
      i. Changes focus of attention away from source of embarrassment
      ii.
   c. ______________________________

Reading 5.2

Nurses' Perceptions of Sexuality Relating to Patient Care

Caitrian Guthrie, MSc, MA, RGN, DipN, DipEd, RNT
Lecturer, School of Nursing & Midwifery, The Robert Gordon University, Aberdeen

A Historical Perspective on Sexuality

A review of the literature relating to sexuality reveals a complex and ill-defined concept. Van Ooijen & Charnock (1994) question whether a history of sexuality can be trusted, given the nature of the elements which comprise it. Thomson & Scott (1995) voice the same concerns, claiming that the main difficulty lies in the fact that various philosophers and social scientists do not share a 'common conception' of their subject matter. Certainly, the works of Freud (1905), Ellis (1913), Kinsey et al. (1948, 1953) and Masters & Johnson (1966, 1970, 1975) all tend to reflect the main cultural, social and intellectual arguments of their time rather than adhering to any fixed definition of what sexuality is.

Prior to the 1970s, research into sexuality was sexology-orientated rather than sexuality-orientated. Parker & Gagnon (1995) suggest that this concentration on biological sex in preference to the wider concept of sexuality fitted with the **positivist,** scientific nature of research at that time. In the 1970s a change of focus appeared. Writers such as Gagnon & Simon (1973) and Foucault (1979) began to suggest that sexuality was culturally and historically specific and, thus, affected by the society in which it existed. **Social deconstructionism,** as advocated by Parker & Gagnon (1995), entails examining the social influences on sexuality and the impact that they have on the way the concept is viewed. The important factor is the manner in which sexuality is perceived by contemporary society.

The views of society are mirrored by the way nursing has dealt with sexuality. Until the 1970s, nursing remained dominated by the medical model of care. Nurses treated sexuality as a physiological concept, and were concerned purely with matters of sexual health rather than a more **abstract** concept encompassing biological, psychological and sociological dimensions (Salvage, 1990). Since then nursing has gradually moved away from the biomedical model towards **holistic** care. As sexuality came to be considered in a wider sense, so nursing too came to see sexuality as something rather more than a biological **construct.**

What Is Sexuality?

Poorman et al. (1991) offer a broad definition of sexuality as "an integral part of the whole person. Human beings are sexual in every way, all the time. To a large extent sexuality determines who we are. It is an integral part of the uniqueness of every person" (p. 633). If we accept that sexuality is an integral component of the individual, then it follows that it needs to be considered when delivering holistic nursing care.

Sexuality can be viewed as a social **phenomenon** that becomes meaningful because we, as individuals, attribute meaning to it. Gagnon & Simon (1973) suggest that one of the reasons biological definitions predominated in the past was because of our "collective blindness and ineptitude" (p. 19) in searching for the meanings people gave to the concept. Savage (1987) goes as far as to claim that the "different meanings given to sexuality, on both a global and personal scale, are endless" (p. 6). Individual nurses may have different perceptions of sexuality from their patients and from other nurses.

Sexuality and Illness

Because sexuality is an integral part of the individual, any illness has the potential to impinge on it. Savage (1987) outlines examples of factors affecting sexuality, for example disease processes, drugs, surgery and radiotherapy, any of which can have a profound effect on a patient. The effect of alterations in sexuality can be very complex because of the interrelated aspects of biology, sociology and psychology which are involved. Such complexity may make it difficult to assess the effect that an illness is having, but should not deter nurses from considering sexuality when caring for patients. "The important issue is for the topic to be on the agenda at all times, and for nurses to realize that sexuality definitely falls within the remit of holistic nursing care" (Van Ooijen & Charnock, 1994, p. 165).

Aims of the Study

The purpose of the study reported in this article was three-fold:

1. to **conceptualize** the phenomenon of sexuality and related factors from the perspective of staff nurses working in acute surgical wards;
2. to attempt to generate theory to explain this phenomenon; and
3. to explore how nurses' perceptions of sexuality might influence the provision of nursing care.

Method

A **qualitative** approach was adopted in the study, using grounded theory as described by Glaser & Strauss (1967). Researchers using **grounded theory** attempt to explain how individuals arrive at the meanings they give to everyday occurrences, through examining the processes which exist within a specific social setting. This study was designed to conceptualize the meanings given to sexuality by nurses in an acute surgical setting and to consider how this affected the patient care they delivered on a daily basis.

The initial sample for a grounded theory study is determined in order to explore the phenomenon where it exists (Chenitz & Swanson, 1986). The sample for this study was drawn from staff nurses working in the surgical directorate of a large teaching hospital. It was a **selective sample,** deliberately chosen in the hope that the participants would be able to inform the research issue. The nurses worked within a context appropriate to the aims of the study. Emerging data suggested that it was appropriate to continue to sample staff nurses working in this area. The sample was a **convenience** one, with staff nurses on duty when the researcher visited the ward being asked to participate. The study was undertaken as part of a Master's degree, and as such had time constraints imposed which led to a limited **sample size.** This could have affected the study if sufficient data had not been forthcoming. In reality, enough data were generated in order to identify and explore the emergence of several themes.

Data Collection

Data were collected through **in-depth interviews.** Such interviews were felt to offer the flexibility essential for grounded theory (Miller, 1995). A broad framework was devised for early interviews, which then changed as data collection progressed. Initial interviews were relatively unfocused. However, data analysis began with the first interview, allowing subsequent interviews to become increasingly focused as themes and categories began to emerge. Strauss & Corbin (1990) warn of the dangers of becoming too focused and thus excluding the discovery of new data. A conscious effort was made by the researcher to allow **informants** to lead the interviews.

In order for the data to be based in the reality of informants, grounded theory requires the researcher to carry out research in the real setting, with the phenomenon being investigated in the context within which it occurs. A quiet room on one of the wards was made available, which allowed the study to be carried out in the clinical area whilst not compromising confidentiality and privacy.

All interviews were tape-recorded, with the permission of **respondents.** Written notes were made following each interview detailing information not available on the tapes, such as non-verbal signs given out by informants through body language and facial expression.

Data Analysis

A total of 10 interviews were conducted in the course of the study. Each taped interview was **transcribed** prior to the next interview being carried out. Data analysis was carried out as suggested by Strauss & Corbin (1990). Level One (open) coding entailed each transcript being examined line by line, with potential categories being noted in the margins. Following each interview, a concept map was developed to represent the information gathered. A large number of codes were generated in this way. See Figure 1 for an example of open coding.

Level Two (axial) coding involved constant comparative analysis, where the coded data were continually compared with data that had emerged from other interviews and clustered according to properties. The concept maps from each interview were compared for this purpose.

Level Three coding identified core themes which had emerged from the data. Three themes were identified at this stage, with the content of later interviews confirming the findings of earlier ones. Fitting each of the identified categories into a discrete theme proved problematic as they were closely interrelated, with each theme impacting heavily on the other two themes. Figure 2 illustrates the process whereby the Level Two categories were subsumed into three themes. These conceptual themes will be used as a framework for the presentation and discussion of the study findings.

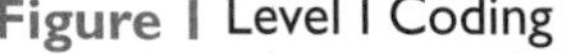
Figure 1 Level 1 Coding

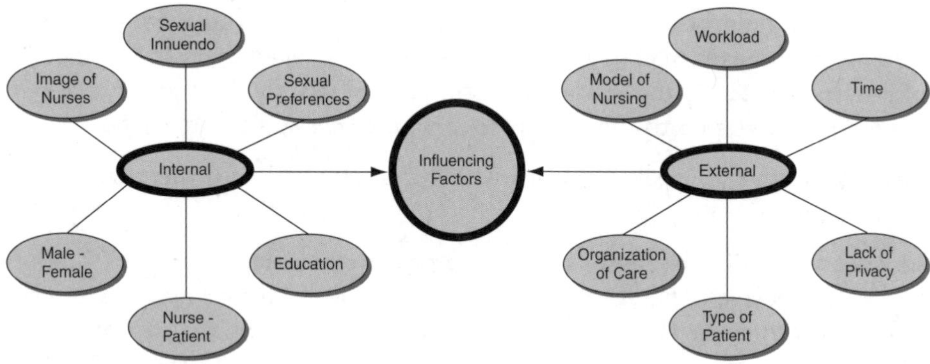

Figure 2 Level II and Level III Coding

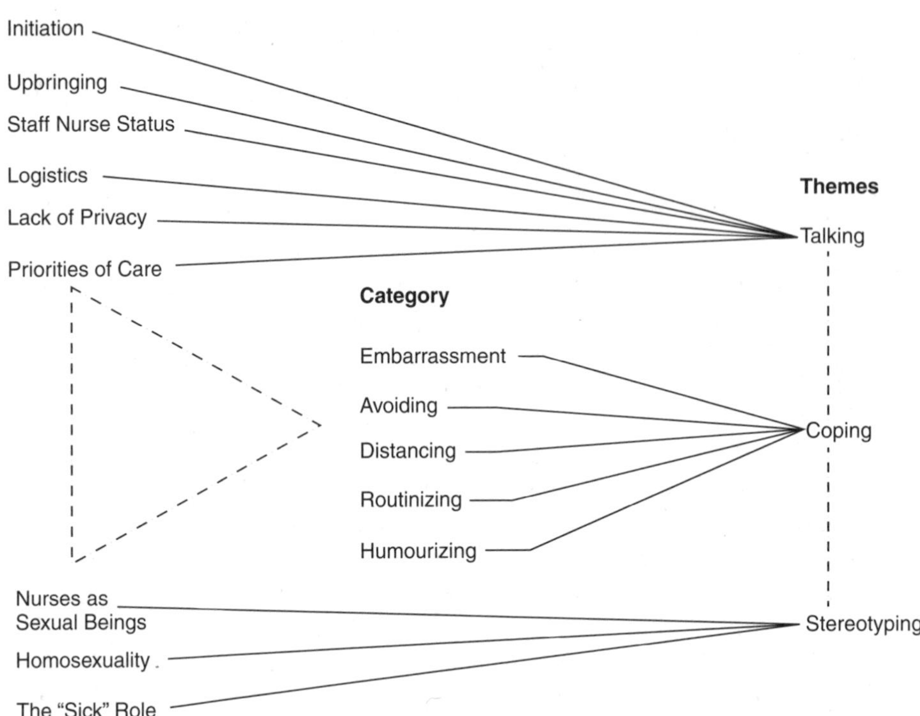

Description and Discussion of Findings

Talking

This theme relates to the process by which information was gained about patient sexuality. Verbal, rather than non-verbal, means of communication were heavily relied upon. It was apparent that, for a variety of reasons, nurses in the study did not generally talk to their patients about sexuality. Respondents felt that it was up to the patient to initiate discussion on sexuality:

> If somebody wanted to speak about it I would chat about it with them, but I wouldn't initiate the conversation.

These nurses are not alone in their unwillingness to broach the subject. Matocha & Waterhouse (1993) found that a high percentage of nurses never assessed sexuality with their patients, despite acknowledging a responsibility to do so. There appeared to be an assumption on the part of respondents that patients do not want to discuss concerns about sexuality with nurses. Waterhouse & Metcalfe (1991), however, despite the self-reported limitations of their study, indicated that 92 percent of the healthy people they sampled thought nurses should discuss sexual matters with clients. It is possible that abdication of responsibility to patients is a means by which nurses can avoid dealing with the issue.

The respondents in the present study felt that patients would introduce sexuality into discussion if they wanted to. This perception may be incorrect. Although their findings cannot be generalized to apply to all hospital patients, studies by Kreuger et al. (1979) and Waterhouse & Metcalfe (1991) suggest that patients prefer nurses to initiate discussion regarding sexual concerns. It may be that while nurses are waiting for patients to introduce the subject, patients are waiting for nurses to do so.

The upbringing of nurses was perceived to make discussion of sexuality difficult. Nettleton (1995) argues that beliefs are "rooted in . . . socio-cultural contexts and that lifestyles are inseparable from the socio-cultural structures in which individuals live out their lives" (p. 37). This ties in with Parker & Gagnon's (1995) assertion that sexuality can only be understood in the context of the culture within which it exists. Several respondents noted that it was not just familial upbringing that affected them, but also exposure to a wider social upbringing:

> When I say my upbringing I don't just mean my mum and dad. I mean when I came away to college and the people I lived with.

Lawler (1991) suggests that sexuality "lies on the margins of what is considered dangerous and potentially polluting" (p. 90). It is not seen as a suitable topic for public discourse. Having been brought up in a society where sexuality is viewed in such a manner, it is not difficult to understand how this may have affected the respondents.

All respondents noted the impact of familial upbringing. Those nurses brought up in a family environment where sexuality was considered a taboo subject had wider societal views reinforced by their parents. One nurse noted that:

> It's the sort of thing you're not really meant to speak about . . . At home my father never spoke about anything and if I walked about the house in a nightie or shorts it was, like, get something on. That does reflect on you in later life.

The attitudes these nurses formed may be particularly strong and difficult to overcome when they are placed in situations where they are forced to confront patient sexuality.

Staff nurse status was felt to prevent nurses establishing close relationships with patients, thus limiting the possibility of sexuality being discussed. The following quote expressed a common view:

> The higher up you go the less contact you have with your patients and it's not really the nurses' fault. It's because they are getting so many other responsibilities put on them. They have to deal with these things first and that is just the way it is.

Nurses felt that talk with their patients was limited to routine topics, for instance drug therapy and discharge arrangements. Morse (1991) describes these types of superficial relationships as "clinical relationships" (p. 458). Respondents seemed to regret being unable to forge closer rapport with their patients. However, talking to patients about nursing tasks rather than more meaningful issues can be a means of diverting attention away from difficult issues such as sexuality and minimizing the discussion that takes place. Macleod Clark (1983) claimed that nurses employed tactics such as these to limit the quality and depth of conversation in order to control it. By acting as they do, nurses in the study may be steering conversation away from sexuality, on to safer ground.

Lack of time and a heavy workload was seen to limit the opportunity for discussion:

> It's so seldom that you get the chance to sit down with patients . . . And sometimes it goes on and on when you do and you think, oh my god, I'm going to be here half an hour and it's like I'm rushing to get finished. That's not ideal either.

When nurses had the opportunity to speak to their patients they felt stressed because of pressure of work and demands on their time. This concurs with the findings of Lewis & Bor (1994), who also attributed failure to discuss sexuality to lack of time and excessive workloads. Jarrett & Payne (1995) claim, however, that even when ward areas are quiet, nurses are unlikely to have one-to-one conversations with their patients. It is impossible to either refute or legitimize the perceptions of nurses in the study that they had too little time and too much work to do. Although these may be valid reasons why they do not talk to patients, they are also an acceptable and easy means of excusing remiss behaviour.

Workload and time permitting, finding somewhere to discuss sexuality was problematic, as this quote illustrates:

> Where would you go to actually speak to somebody about it? I don't think it's a good place to speak to somebody if you've just got a curtain between you and the ward.

Lewis & Bor's (1994) study also identified lack of privacy as a reason for not discussing sexuality with patients. There can be little doubt that it is difficult to maintain privacy in an acute ward. However, only one respondent noted making specific efforts to maintain privacy, albeit unsuccessfully. Waterhouse & Metcalfe (1991) suggest that this lack of privacy adds to problems in patients who already feel "asexual" as a result of invasive procedures, medication side-effects and limited visiting hours.

Respondents claimed that patient sexuality was not discussed in the acute surgical setting because it was not a priority of care. As seen in this comment, physical problems were seen to take precedence:

> You are so concerned about the other problems they are coming in with that you're not really concerned with sexuality.

Kautz et al. (1990) also concluded that nurses saw the sexual concerns of their patients as a low priority. Such claims could be dismissed as a means of avoiding the issue, but they may be valid. A study of hospitalized patients, including general surgical patients, by Von Essen & Sjoden (1991) found that patients want their nurses to be technically competent and are more concerned with physical than psychological care. It could be argued, however, that although there are certain surgical patients for whom sexuality might not be an overwhelming concern, there may equally be surgical patients for whom it is very much an issue. Unless nurses are willing to introduce the topic, they will be unable to assess the patient's needs regarding sexuality. If a patient does not wish to pursue the issue then this has to be respected, but the opportunity for discussion needs to be available.

Stereotyping

The theme of stereotyping revealed that respondents perceived the public to hold stereotyped ideas of nurses, and also that nurses themselves held stereotyped ideas about certain groups of patients. These stereotypes were closely interrelated with gender issues. Fiske et al. (1993) claim that such stereotypes tend to be prescriptive and powerful because of the early and repeated exposure that individuals have to these stereotypes.

Nurses perceived the public image of nurses to be that of sex objects, and they attributed this to the way nurses are portrayed in the media. As one respondent suggested:

> There's always a stigma attached to a nurse, isn't there? I mean, all the comedy acts and all you see is the nurse with stockings and the high-heeled shoes and massive boobs.

These nurses are not alone in their perception that the media impinges on images that people have of nurses. Kalisch & Kalisch (1982,1983) demonstrated that the media has a strong effect on public views and claimed that constant misrepresentation of nurses results in negative image formation by the public. Respondents were very definite in their perception that the public derived sexual connotations from their role. This stereotyping affected the way nurses perceived patient behaviour towards them. One nurse suggested that:

> They [the patients] like to think of you as this stereotyped nurse with the short skirt and the suspenders. . . .

This affected the way they perceived patient behaviour towards them.

Webb (1985) suggests that the most "visible intrusion" of sexual stereotyping into nursing is the uniform. Respondents wore traditional, white dresses. White represents purity and fits in with the idea of nurse as angel. Szasz et al. (1982) claim that this very whiteness can be sexually arousing for males. Respondents' uniforms were also see-through and thus provocative. Male patients were noted to have reacted to this:

> They say the usual things, like "You can see your pants through your skirt" ... one spoke about the Panty Parade. Every nurse that went past we realized he could see through her uniform.

This type of uniform actively encourages a view of nurses as sexual beings. A change to functional, rather than decorative, uniforms might help dispel the myth of nurses as sexual objects.

All 10 nurses interviewed reported having been exposed to sexual harassment. One respondent described patient behaviour:

> They'll pinch your bum, but I'm glad to say that doesn't happen very often. Occasionally you will get them doing things like that or they will say things like "You're a big girl" and they have a look at your chest....

Despite self-reported limitations, a study by Finnis & Robbins (1994) claimed that a high percentage of female nurses had experienced sexual harassment. This confirmed the findings of previous studies (Grieco, 1987; Finnis et al., 1993). They also found the main perpetrators to be hospital patients.

This may be linked not only to stereotypes of female nurses as sex objects, but also to common male stereotypes. Henley & Freeman (1982) state that "social interaction is where the daily war between the sexes is fought" (p. 83). The social interactions that take place between nurses and patients are often atypical, forcing the male into a non-dominant role. When nurses in the study gave patients suppositories, as they frequently did, they held the power. One nurse commented:

> When they see me coming with their Voltarol suppositories, then they know who's the boss!

Not only were male patients asked to expose taboo parts of their bodies, but they were also subjected to a level of intimacy not normally found in an interaction between relative strangers. Porter (1995) suggests that one way the male can counter this demeaning of his image and intrusion of his body is by demeaning the nurse in return. This can be achieved through sexual harassment.

The sexual harassment reported by respondents may be caused by misinterpretations of the nurse-patient relationship by patients. Much of nurses' work involves touch. Lawler (1991) claims that men see such touch as sexual. Fagin & Diets (1984) assert that nursing is a "metaphor for sex" (p. 17), contending that because of this metaphor and because nurses so often touch their male patients, patients perceive them as willing to enter into sexual interactions. Nurses use touch so routinely in their everyday work that it is doubtful whether it has the same meaning to them. As one nurse pointed out:

> We are so used to touching people, to touching people all over their bodies, that we just don't think anything of it. It's just part of our job.

Johnson et al. (1991) found that men were more liable to view male-female interaction in a sexual way than women. Perhaps male patients, perceived by nurses in the study to be perpetrators of sexual harassment, had misinterpreted the relationship in this way.

Another feature of perceived sexual harassment was that nurses appeared to be accepting as long as it was mild, although one respondent questioned whether they should:

> I think female nurses accept it, but I don't think they should ... If it is once then that is fair enough, but if it is more than once it does affect your overall care.

The stereotyped public image of nurses as sex objects accepted by these nurses, along with stereotyped images of the male patient, might explain this. If harassment can be blamed on nurses as an occupational group and male behaviour in general, then the nurses need not personalize these incidents. Such logic makes it easier for the nurses to cope with the sexual harassment they are subjected to.

Sexual stereotyping also led to difficulties when caring for homosexual patients and attitudes of nurses to homosexuals were negative:

> I think there is still a stigma attached to that sort of thing. If you were to write down [on the assessment sheet] gay man or something, I think there would be this sort of stigma attached. It's terrible, but there it is.

Research carried out by Siminoff et al. (1991) indicates that some female nurses do have negative attitudes towards homosexuals. Although some respondents felt nursing care was affected only transiently, even initial, short-lived reactions to a patient's sexuality might impact quite severely on that particular patient.

Homosexual males might be considered deviant—that is, not conforming to expected norms—as a "collective denial of the social order" (Goffman, 1963, p. 171). Rafferty (1995) suggests that society determines what is "normal" and "healthy" by setting up codes of moral values. She claims that nursing, which has historically been a conservative occupation, has readily embraced these societal norms and thus stereotyped images of homosexuals as deviant and bad have flourished within nursing.

Nurses in the study perceived the care given to homosexual patients as inadequate, and expressed concerns about this. One nurse described the reactions of other staff when a homosexual man was admitted to her ward:

> People were saying things like "I'm not touching him, I'm not going near him." I thought that was pretty bad, considering we're meant to be a caring profession.

Dissonance occurred when nurses, who recognized that they were bound by their professional code to care, were unable to do so because of their own attitudes and beliefs. The main way of overcoming this dissonance was to avoid talking to homosexual patients about their sexuality.

Coping

Previous themes dealt with factors that respondents identified as affecting patient care in relation to sexuality. The focus of this theme is different, as it considers ways in which nurses coped with issues that emerged in the preceding themes.

Although the category of embarrassment does not fit neatly into this theme, it emerged as an antecedent to all the coping strategies employed and will therefore be presented and discussed within this theme. Edelmann (1981) claims that embarrassment can be attributed "to the violation of social expectations which govern and define desirable behaviour" (p. 126). Nurses in this study became embarrassed when either they or others behaved in ways perceived to fall outside these accepted behaviours. Respondents noted high levels of embarrassment when performing intimate, sometimes invasive procedures:

> Things like giving young guys suppositories, that's embarrassing. I don't like doing that.

Embarrassment often involves instances where privacy has been breached. Lawler (1991) suggests that this is an important aspect in nurses' construction of the concept. Breaches of privacy occur when nurses touch or come too close to patients, or when a taboo part of the body is exposed.

Embarrassment on the part of a nurse when suppositories were given indicates that the nurse realized that she had broken the normal rules of bodily intimacy.

Events which are given inappropriate sexual connotations can also cause embarrassment. Both nurses and patients were reported in the study as ascribing inappropriate meanings to routine care. Nurses reported embarrassment when caring for homosexual patients, yet the routine care of these patients should be no different from that of any other patient. Embarrassment was the result of nurses reading sexual meanings into situations which were no different from other everyday happenings. Several respondents noted that they felt embarrassed because a patient was embarrassed:

> If the patient is embarrassed then I do tend to get embarrassed because I feel their embarrassment.

Edelman (1981) calls this "vicarious embarrassment." Lawler (1991) suggests that nurses have to learn to manage these situations effectively: not showing discomfort gives the patient permission not to be embarrassed either.

Respondents employed various strategies in order to cope with embarrassment. Benner and Wrubel (1989) suggest that coping possibilities depend on the context within which an event occurs. Nurses, because of their duty of care, have limited means of coping. Avoidance and distancing are two options available to them. Valentine (1995) claims that avoidance is the most common tactic employed by nurses when faced with potentially confrontational situations. The nurses in this study admitted using avoidance on a regular basis:

> You do avoid things very often. You brush over things . . . you brush over sexuality a lot.

Rather than deal with the perpetrators of sexual innuendos, nurses either avoided them or distanced themselves. The issue did not then need to be confronted.

Avoidance and distancing can be seen in the light of the complex nurse-patient relationship. The nurse wields considerable power in this relationship (Lowenberg, 1994). By avoiding patients and distancing themselves, nurses asserted their power. Wiley (1987) calls this "coercive power." Negative sanctions, which detracted from the standard of care offered, were put in place, and unless the patient behaved in an acceptable manner, these sanctions remained in place:

> You make sure that they get their medication, that they get their meals, that they get whatever it is . . . and then you smile sweetly and walk off.

Routinizing behaviour took place where breaches of privacy had occurred. Respondents attempted to alleviate patient embarrassment by claiming that the event causing the emotion was routine and everyday to them. By minimizing the situation in this way, nurses were employing what Lawler (1991) termed "minifisms." She defined these as "verbal and/or behavioural techniques which assist in the management of potentially problematic situations by minimising the size, significance or severity of an event involving a patient" (p. 166). One nurse reported how she dealt with giving painkilling suppositories to a young male patient:

> I'm a bit abrupt really. I tell them it's nothing, just a pain killer and I'm going to go out of here and not think any more of it.

Such routinizing helped both patients and nurses cope.

A final coping mechanism identified was use of humour. Sometimes this was at the expense of the patient, as demonstrated below, where a nurse describes the reaction of nursing staff to comments made by patients when filling in the "Expressing Sexuality" component of the admission sheet used in her clinical area:

> If the patient writes anything we'll look at it and say "Look at that, they're still doing it at their age!" You laugh about it....

More often, humour was shared with patients during embarrassing situations. Nurses may have been engaged in what Edelman (1987) terms "face-saving," where humour is used to change the focus of attention and divert it away from the cause of embarrassment. An embarrassed patient becomes an equal participant in the interaction, rather than the victim of an embarrassing event. Respondents also rationalized the behaviour of patients, excusing inappropriate use of humour as a means of coping with embarrassment.

Conclusions and Recommendations

This study was both small and localized. The perceptions of respondents and the context within which they occurred are unique and the findings cannot be generalized to any other population of staff nurses. However, the results may cause other nurses to reflect upon their own practice.

The overall conclusion is that the nurses studied find it problematic to provide nursing care relating to sexuality. They are unwilling to introduce sexuality as a facet of patient care for a variety of reasons, some contextual, some residual. Nurses need to examine the reasons why they are so reluctant to talk about sexuality with patients. It would be extremely difficult to change societal attitudes towards homosexuality. However, nurses must be encouraged to examine their attitudes, both individually and collectively, and to gain insight into their own behaviour and that of their peers. This could be achieved through the organization of discussion forums within clinical areas.

Equally difficult to bring about would be a change in the way nurses are portrayed as sex objects in the media. A concerted effort on the part of the nursing profession is needed to put pressure on those elements of the media that continue to reinforce this image. Hospital policies relating to sexual harassment should be openly displayed and made available to nurses. Assertiveness training should be offered to those nurses who require it.

Introducing sexuality as part of the nursing curriculum is of little use if nurses cannot integrate such theory into practice. Education should be geared not only towards providing nurses with knowledge about sexuality, but also to equipping them with the communication skills necessary to operationalize that knowledge.

Issues such as sexuality will only be discussed openly if the setting is conducive to this. Private areas need to be set aside where nurses and patients can discuss sexuality without fear of being interrupted or overheard. These areas would be of benefit not only for talking about sexuality, but also for discussion of any topic that requires privacy.

If these recommendations are implemented, then it is possible that the provision of patient care relating to sexuality will improve. The ability to provide more holistic care for patients should enhance the self-esteem not only of the patient, but also of the nurse.

References

Benner P., & Wrubel J. (1989). *The primacy of caring: Stress and coping in health and illness.* San Francisco: Addison-Wesley.

Chenitz, W. C., & Swanson, J. M. (1986). *From practice to grounded theory.* San Francisco: Addison-Wesley.

Edelmann, R. J. (1981). Embarrassment: The state of research. *Current Psychological Reviews 1981, 1,* 125–138.

———. (1987). *The psychology of embarrassment.* Chichester, UK: Wiley.

Ellis, H. (1913). *Studies in the psychology of sex,* Vols 1–6. Philadelphia: Davis.

Fagin, C., & Diers, D. (1984). Nursing as metaphor. *International Nursing Review 31*(1), 16–17.

Finnis S. J., & Robbins, I. (1994). Sexual harassment of nurses: An occupational hazard? *Journal of Clinical Nursing 3,* 87–95.

Finnis, S., Robbins, I., & Bender, M. P. (1993). A pilot study of the prevalence and psychological sequelae of sexual harassment of nursing staff. *Journal of Clinical Nursing 2,* 23–27.

Fiske, S. T., & Stevens, L. E. (1993). What's so special about sex? In S. Oskamp & M. Costanzo (Eds.), *Gender issues in contemporary society* (pp. 173–196). Newbury Park: Sage.

Foucault, M. (1979). *History of Sexuality,* Vol. 1. London: Allen Lane.

Freud, S. (1905). *Three essays on theory of sexuality.* London: Hogarth.

Gagnon, J., & Simon, W. (1973). *Sexual construct: The social sources of human sexuality.* Chicago: Aldine.

Glaser, B. G., & Strauss, A. L. (1967). *The discovery of grounded theory: Strategies for qualitative research.* London: Aldine.

Goffman, E. (1963). *Stigma: Notes on the management or a spoiled identity.* London: Penguin.

Grieco, A. (1987). The scope and nature of sexual harassment in nursing. *Journal of Sex Research 23*(2), 261–266.

Johnson, C. B., Stockdale, M. S., & Saal, F. E. (1991). Persistence of men's misconceptions of friendly cues across a variety of interpersonal encounters. *Psychology of Women Quarterly 15,* 463–475.

Kalisch, P. A., & Kalisch, B. J. (1982, Feb.). Nurses on prime-time television. *American Journal of Nursing,* 264–270.

———. (1983, Jan.). Improving the image of nursing. *American Journal of Nursing,* 48–52.

Kautz, D. D., Dickey, C. A., & Stevens, M. N. (1990). Using research to identify why nurses do not meet established sexuality nursing care standards. *Journal of Nursing Quality Assurance 4*(3), 69–78.

Kinsey, A., Pomeroy, W. B., & Martin, C. E. (1948). *Sexual behavior in the human male.* Philadelphia: Saunders.

———. (1953). *Sexual behavior in the human female.* Philadelphia: Saunders.

Kreuger, J. C., Hassel, J., Goggins, B. B., Ishimatso, T., Pablico, M. R., & Tuttle, E. J. (1979). Relationship between nurse counseling and sexual adjustment after hysterectomy. *Nursing Research 28,* 145–150.

Lawler J. (1991). *Behind the screens: Nursing, somology and the problem of the body.* Melbourne: Churchill Livingstone.

Lewis, S. L., & Bor, R. (1994). Nurses' knowledge of and attitudes towards sexuality and the relationship of these with nursing practice. *Journal of Advanced Nursing 20,* 251–259.

Lowenberg, J. G. (1994). The nurse-patient relationship reconsidered: An expanded research agenda. *Image: Scholarly inquiry for nursing practice 8*(2), 167–184.

Macleod Clark, J. (1983). Nurse-patient communication—an analysis of conversations from surgical wards. In J. Wilson-Barnett (Ed.), *Nursing Research Ten Studies in Patient Care.* Chichester, UK: Wiley.

Masters, W., & Johnson, V. (1966). *Human sexual response.* Boston: Little, Brown & Co.

———. (1970). *Human sexual response.* Boston: Little, Brown & Co.

———. (1975). *The pleasure bond.* Boston: Little, Brown & Co.

Matocha, L. K., & Waterhouse, J. K. (1993). Current nursing practice related to sexuality. *Research in Nursing and Health 16,* 371–378.

Morse, J. M. (1991). Negotiating commitment and involvement in the nurse-patient relationship. *Journal of Advanced Nursing 16,* 455–468.

Nettleton, S. (1995). *The sociology of health and illness.* Cambridge: Polity.

Parker, R. G., & Gagnon, J.H. (1995). *Conceiving sexuality.* New York: Routledge.

Poorman, S. (1991). Variations in sexual response. In G. Stuart & S. Sundeen (Eds.), *Principles and practice of psychiatric nursing* (4th ed.). St. Louis: Mosby.

Porter, S. (1995). Women in a women's job: The gendered experience of nurses. *Sociology of Health and Illness 14*(4), 510–521.

Rafferty, D. (1995). Putting sexuality on the agenda. *Nursing Times 91*(17), 28–31.

Salvage, J. (1990). Theory and practice of the 'new nursing.' *Nursing Times 86*(4), 42–45.

Savage J. (1987). *Nurses, gender and sexuality.* London: Heinemann.

Siminoff, L. A., Erlin, J. A., & Lidz, C. W. (1991). Stigma, AIDS and quality of nursing care: State of the science. *Journal of Advanced Nursing 16,* 262–269.

Strauss, A., & Corbin, J. (1990). *Basics of qualitative research: Grounded theory procedures and techniques.* Newbury Park: Sage.

Szasz, S., in Muff, J. (Ed.) (1982). *Socialization, sexism and stereotyping: Women's issues in nursing.* St. Louis: Mosby.

Thomson, R., & Scott, S. (1995). *Researching sexuality in the light of AIDS: Historical and methodological issues.* London: Tufnell.

Valentine, P. E. B. (1995). Management of conflict: Do nurses/women handle it differently? *Journal of Advanced Nursing 22,* 142–149.

Van Ooijen, E., & Charnock, A. (1994). *Sexuality and patient care: A guide for nurses and teachers.* London: Chapman Hall.

Von Essen, L., & Sjoden, P. (1991). The importance of nurse caring behaviours as perceived by Swedish hospital patients and nursing staff. *International Journal of Nursing Studies 28*(3), 267–281.

Waterhouse, J., & Metcalfe, M. (1991). Attitudes toward nurses discussing sexual concerns with patients. *Journal of Advanced Nursing 16,* 1048–1054.

Webb, C. (1985). *Sexuality, nursing and health.* Chichester, UK: Wiley.

———. (1988). A study of nurses' knowledge and attitudes about sexuality in health care. *International Journal of Nursing Studies 25*(3), 235–244.

Wiley, E. L. (1987). Acquiring and using power effectively. *Journal of Continuing Education in Nursing 18*(1), 25–27.

Comprehension and Discussion Questions

The questions ask you to locate important information in the reading, as well as respond to some of the issues discussed in the article from both a personal and cultural perspective.

1. On page 183, the author claims that "prior to the 1970s, research into sexuality was sexology-orientated rather than sexuality-orientated." Reread the introduction, in particular the last three paragraphs. Make a list of the concepts, terms, and phrases that are used to explain these two different perspectives, both in society in general, as well as in nursing.
2. Why should sexuality be considered part of the holistic care of individuals?
3. What are the different ways in which nurses avoid *talking* about sexuality with patients?
4. On page 189, the author claims that "[sexual harassment] may be linked not only to stereotypes of female nurses as sex objects, but also to common male stereotypes." What are the common male stereotypes that are routinely challenged in an acute health-care setting?
5. How do male patients and female nurses view touch? How might different perceptions of touch lead to sexual harassment?
6. On page 189, one nurse states in response to sexual harassment: "I think female nurses accept it, but I don't think they should . . . If it is once then that is fair enough, but if it is more than once it does affect your overall care." How would you respond if you were sexually harassed by a client? Do you think a nurse should accept it if it happens only once? Why or why not? How do you think sexual harassment could affect overall care of a client?
7. How does your culture view sexual harassment? How does your culture respond to sexual harassment? Do you agree or disagree with your culture's perception of and response to sexual harassment? Why or why not?
8. How do negative attitudes toward gays and lesbians affect patient care? Do you have certain beliefs about homosexuality that could affect your attitude and behavior toward gay and lesbian patients? If so, how will you fulfill your professional responsibility to provide quality care to all individuals?
9. What are the author's recommendations for improving the provision of patient care relating to sexuality?
10. What do you think are the greatest barriers for nurses from your cultural background providing patient care related to sexuality? What recommendations do you have for reducing those barriers for yourself and others from your cultural background?

Research Terminology

Reading 5.2 contains many words about qualitative research design and analysis.

Activity: Understanding Research Terminology

Research Design and Analysis

Match each word about research design and analysis with its definition.

a. positivism
b. social constructivism
c. abstract
d. holistic
e. construct
f. grounded theory
g. selective sample
h. convenience sample
i. sample size
j. in-depth interviews
k. informants
l. respondents
m. transcribe
n. phenomenon
o. conceptualize
p. qualitative

1. ____________________:
   To form an idea about something.
2. ____________________:
   Participants that are selected for a study because they meet a certain criteria, usually their knowledge about the subject of inquiry.
3. ____________________:
   Existing only as an idea or quality rather than as something real that you can see or touch.
4. ____________________:
   A belief system that claims there is an objective reality or truth that can be discovered through systematic inquiry into cause-and-effect relationships.
5. ____________________:
   Method of treatment involving all the patients' mental and family circumstances rather than just dealing with the condition from which he or she is suffering.
6. ____________________:
   The number of participants in a study.
7. ____________________:
   The actual characteristic or ability in a human being.
8. ____________________:
   The means of gathering information or data from participants in a study in which the interviewer encourages informants to reveal the knowledge they possess, rather than to respond to narrowly focused questions that presuppose certain kinds of answers.

9. ____________________:
Interpretation of data in ethnographic research that is based on discovering the patterns and relationships in the data, or from the ground up.

10. ____________________:
To write something down exactly as it was said, in research, usually from a recording of an interview.

11. ____________________:
Something that happens or exists in society, science, or nature, often something that people discuss or study because it is difficult to understand.

12. ____________________:
A belief system that claims there is no objective reality, but rather mental constructions of phenomena. Truth is arrived at through consensus among people.

13. ____________________:
Participants in a study that responded to an instrument of some kind, like a questionnaire.

14. ____________________:
Participants in a study who are particularly well informed about the subject of inquiry, articulate, approachable, or available.

15. ____________________:
An approach to research that does not quantify the results into preexisting categories of analysis, but rather allows the categories of analysis to emerge from the data and represents the findings in words, not numbers.

16. ____________________:
Participants that were selected for their availability or accessibility.

Journal Entry: Reflecting on Sexuality in Nursing

Write two to three pages synthesizing and reflecting on what you have learned from the two readings about sexuality in nursing. Answer the questions:

1. In general, what have you learned about sexuality in nursing from the readings?
2. Has your understanding and attitude toward sexuality in nursing changed as a result of the readings? If so, how?
3. What concerns do you have as a nurse in assessing, treating, and teaching clients about sexuality?

UNIT

6

Ethical Dilemmas in Nursing

The **content-based objectives** include understanding and thinking critically about

- Female circumcision, the main types, short- and long-term complications, and the reason why it is practiced
- Principles of autonomy, patient rights, informed consent, cultural relativism, and cultural competence as they relate to a discussion of the legal and ethical implications of female circumcision in the United States
- End-of-life issues from a cross-cultural perspective
  The principles of autonomy, beneficence, veracity, truth disclosure, informed consent, and community as they relate to a discussion of truth disclosure of a terminal illness

The **skill-based objectives** include

- Applying critical reading skills to the reading of two articles about ethical dilemmas
- Integrating information from the two articles into your writing about ethical dilemmas in nursing
- Thinking critically about the ethical issues posed by female circumcision and truth disclosure

Ethical Issues: A Cross-Cultural Perspective

Clients and health care providers do not always share the same beliefs, values, and practices with regard to health care, especially when they do not share the same cultural background. Such differences can lead to ethical dilemmas. An **ethical dilemma** is a situation that can arise due to a conflict in values about what is right or wrong or differences in the understanding of rights and responsibilities.

Health care professionals are guided by the principle of **beneficence**, or "doing good" for the patient. The rights of patients are protected by the principle of **patient autonomy** or the right of patients to make their own decisions with regard to their own health care. **Cultural relativism** recognizes the equality of all cultures.

What happens when these principles come into conflict? This unit will examine ethical issues raised by the cultural practice of female circumcision and cultural practices regarding end-of-life issues. In addition to mental health and illness and sexuality, female circumcision and end-of-life issues are difficult topics for many international and immigrant students to discuss. Early exposure to these topics will help students think about these issues from multiple perspectives and become more comfortable talking about them before they encounter them in their nursing programs. Also, because of increased immigration from countries where female circumcision is widely practiced, female circumcision is an important issue for nursing students to understand, not only from a health care perspective, but also from a cultural and ethical one. Nurses provide health care for circumcised women and girls and need to know not only what it is and the medical complications of this practice, but also the cultural, legal, and ethical implications.

Female Circumcision

Female circumcision, also referred to as female genital mutilation or FGM, refers to a "group of traditional practices that involve partial or total removal of the external female genitalia or other injury to the female genital organs for cultural, religious, or other non-therapeutic reasons (Jones, Smith, Kieke, & Wilcox, 1997, p. 1). There are estimated to be 27 countries in the world with prevalence rates from 5 to 99 percent—that is, at least 5 percent of the girls and women and up to 99 percent of the girls and women in these countries undergo some type of circumcision (Toubia, 1994). Although this practice is found in some countries in Southeast Asia and the Middle East, most of the countries that practice female circumcision are in Africa.

The number of immigrants to the United States from countries in Africa increased by 99 percent from 192,300 in 1981–1990 to 383,000 in 1991–2000, an increase of 190,700 (U.S. Census Bureau, 2004a). In addition, the number of refugees admitted from countries that practice female circumcision has also increased, most notably from Somalia, Ethiopia, Sudan, and Liberia (U.S. Census Bureau, 2004b). The prevalence rate of female circumcision in these countries is 98, 90, 89, and 60 percent, respectively (Toubia, 1994).

Pre-Reading Activity

Discuss in small groups your answers to these questions. Form groups with classmates who do not have the same cultural background.

1. Give an example of a cultural practice in your community that conflicts with mainstream culture in the United States. Explain what it is and why it conflicts with U.S. culture.
2. Give an example of a cultural practice in your community that has changed since you or your family came to the United States. How has it changed and why?
3. Give an example of a cultural practice that has *not* changed. Why has it not changed?
4. Are there some practices that are easier to give up or change than others? Why?

Reading about Female Circumcision

To read about female circumcision, locate and read this article in your university or college library:

Gibeau, A. M. (1998). Female genital mutilation: When a cultural practice generates clinical and ethical dilemmas. *Journal of Obstetric, Gynecologic, & Neonatal Nursing, 27,* 85–91.

This article not only provides information about the practice of female circumcision, but it also discusses the legal and ethical issues posed by the practice in the United States. Ethical principles that are discussed in the article include: autonomy, patient rights, informed consent, cultural relativism, and cultural competence.

Activity: Understanding Ethical Principles

Match each ethical principle with its definition.

a. autonomy
b. patient rights
c. informed consent
d. cultural relativism
e. cultural competence

1. ____________________:
The belief that all cultures are inherently equal and that all customs within a particular culture make sense within the context of that culture.

2. ____________________:
The ability of rational beings to make choices based on accurate information.

3. ____________________:
An approach to the delivery of health care that takes into consideration the total context of the client's situation and requires the health care provider to use a combination of knowledge, attitudes, and skills

4. ____________________:
The right of patients to make autonomous decisions about medical treatment, including the right to refuse treatment.

5. ____________________:
The decision approving medical treatment that a patient makes after having been given all the information he or she needs to make a rational decision about that treatment

Activity: Vocabulary Development

Select 15–20 words from the article that you do not know. These words should be words associated with main ideas, not details, in the article. Add these words to your dictionary, following the guidelines on page 33. Use a medical English dictionary to look up medical/nursing terms and a college-level English dictionary to look up socio-cultural terms that you do not know. Use as many of these words as you can in your responses to the questions that follow.

Comprehension and Discussion Questions

The questions ask you to locate important information in the reading, as well as analyze carefully and think critically about the issues raised in this article. The page numbers given apply to those in the reading (not provided) and do not refer to pages in this book. Discuss your answers in small groups.

1. What is female circumcision or female genital mutilation (FGM)? How many types of female circumcision are there? Describe each one.

2. Why is female circumcision practiced? List the reasons that are given in the article. Are there other reasons you could add to this list? In your opinion, which of these reasons is the most important? Why? The least important? Why?

3. What are the immediate and long-term complications of female circumcision?

4. Do you agree that female circumcision is similar to such practices as breast augmentation and liposuction? Why or why not?

5. On page 87, the author states: "One misconception among health care providers is that the FGM seen in émigrés was performed in their home countries. This misconception is important to correct because there is evidence that FGM continues to be practiced among immigrant populations in their new countries, possibly including the United States." Do you think the practice of female circumcision in immigrant communities will diminish over time or will it continue to be practiced, even among subsequent generations? Explain your answer.

6. On page 88, the author claims that "most affected women [who have experienced FGM] do not attribute their health problems to FGM." Why are affected women not more aware of the health-related complications of FGM?

7. Why have efforts to eradicate FGM failed? In your opinion, what would be the most effective way to eradicate this practice?

8. In what ways are autonomy and patient rights challenged when providing culturally competent care to women from cultures where FGM is practiced?

9. Why does Schwartz argue that "consent for any form of FGM by adult women cannot be given freely" (page 90). Do you agree or disagree with this claim? Explain your answer.

10. Why is cultural relativism important in a discussion of culturally competent care of women from cultures where FGM is practiced?

Journal Entry: Ethical Dilemma 1

You are a nurse midwife taking care of a Somali client who has just given birth to her first child. She was infibulated and in order to allow for normal delivery of the baby, you performed a dual episiotomy (with both posterior and anterior cuts). What would you do as a follow-up to the episiotomy? The normal procedure for a regular (posterior) episiotomy is to sew the cut, but for the anterior cut, what would you do? Would you just suture the edges or would you sew her back up as she was before with the urethea and vagina covered (re-infibulation)? Would you refuse to do it even if she asks you to? Why? What options would you offer her?

Your response should discuss the cultural and ethical dilemma posed by re-infibulation, including reference to the concepts of autonomy, patient rights, informed consent, cultural relativity, and cultural competence. Your answer should include information from the reading about the cultural practice of circumcision, as well as health risks associated with infibulation and re-infibulation. Your entry should be two to three pages.

Discuss your responses to this dilemma in small groups.

End-of-Life Issues

Different cultural perspectives about end-of-life issues also can raise ethical dilemmas for nurses. A close examination of the principles that are used in North America to help patients make decisions regarding treatment for terminal illness are based on **individual autonomy**—the right of the individual to know and to make his or her own decisions. In most other cultures around the world and even within minority cultures in the United States, the family is the locus of decision-making. It is the family, not the individual, who takes responsibility for end-of-life issues.

In addition, there are fundamentally different interpretations of the principle of **beneficence.** In bioethics, nurses are obligated "to implement actions that benefit clients and support persons" (Kozier, Erb, Blais, & Wilkinson, 1995, p. 168). But, what does it mean to "do good"? In most cultures around the world, it would be considered cruel to tell someone they have a terminal illness. In the United States, it is considered unethical **not** to tell a patient the truth about his or her prognosis.

Pre-Reading Activity

Discuss in small groups your answers to these questions. Form groups with classmates who do not have the same cultural background.

1. How is death and dying viewed and handled in your culture?
2. How comfortable are you talking about death and dying?
3. What difficulties do you anticipate as a nurse working with patients who are dying?

Reading about End-of-Life Issues

To read about end-of-life issues from a cross-cultural perspective, locate and read this article in your university or college library:

Lapine, A., Wang-Cheng, R., Goldstein, M., Nooney, A., Lamb, G., & Derse, A. R. (2001). When cultures clash: Physician, patient, and family wishes in truth disclosure fordying patients. *Journal of Palliative Medicine, 4*, 475–480.

This article describes two clinical case studies in which the families of patients with terminal illness did not wish the patient to be informed about the truth of his condition, thus challenging the principle of patient autonomy. In the first case the family is Chinese and in the second case Georgian.

Activity: Understanding Ethical Principles

Match each ethical principle with its definition.

a. autonomy
b. beneficence
c. moral absolutism
d. veracity
e. truth disclosure
f. moral relativism
g. informed consent
h. community

1. ____________________:
The needs of the group, often the family unit, are considered more important than the needs of the individual.

2. ____________________:
The belief that what is right and what is wrong are fixed and do not change from one situation or context to another.

3. ____________________:
Telling the truth about a patient's diagnosis and prognosis for treatment and recovery.

4. ____________________:
The decision approving medical treatment that a patient makes after having been given all the information needed to make a rational decision about that treatment.

5. ____________________:
The belief that what is right and wrong are not fixed and do change from one situation or context to another.

6. ____________________:
The ability of rational beings to make choices based on accurate information.

7. ____________________:
The mandate of the physician and other health care providers to act for the good of the patient.

8. ____________________:
Truthfulness.

Activity: Vocabulary Development

Select 15–20 words from the article that you do not know. These words should be words associated with main ideas, not details, in the article. Add these words to your dictionary, following the guidelines on page 33. Use a medical English dictionary to look up medical/nursing terms and a college-level English dictionary to look up ethical concepts/principles and cultural values/concepts that you do not know. Use as many of these words as you can in your responses to the questions that follow.

Comprehension and Discussion Questions

The questions ask you to locate important information in the reading, as well as analyze carefully and think critically about the issues raised in the article.

1. Why is patient autonomy so important in the United States? Why is patient autonomy a potential source of conflict in providing care for patients with a terminal illness who are not from mainstream U.S. culture?
2. In the case of the 71-year-old gentleman from China, why did the resident want to tell the patient the truth about his diagnosis?
3. In the case of the Chinese patient, why did the family not want the biopsy done? Why did the family not want the patient told the truth about his diagnosis? What Chinese cultural values explain the family's behavior in both refusing the biopsy and in shielding the patient from the truth?
4. In the case of the Chinese patient, what compromise did the Ethics Committee propose? In your opinion, was the compromise successful? Why or why not?
5. The wife of the 47-year-old gentleman from the Republic of Georgia also requested that her husband not be told the truth about his diagnosis. What were the reasons she gave?
6. What Georgian cultural values explain not only the wife's decision not to tell her husband, but also her husband's willingness to have his wife make medical decisions for him? What other reasons were given that also help to explain this decision?
7. What compromise did the Ethics Committee propose in the case of the Georgian patient? How did it differ from the compromise proposed in the case of the Chinese patient? In your opinion, was the compromise successful? Why or why not?
8. The authors argue that the concept of autonomy should be reexamined. What do they propose for a new definition? Do you agree with this reformulation? Why or why not?

9. Look at the questions in Table 2 in the reading (not provided). As a future health care provider, would you be comfortable with asking a terminally ill patient these questions? Are there any questions you would change or add?

10. Look at the suggestions in Table 1 in the reading (not provided) for dealing with cultural conflicts. Are there any suggestions you would change or add?

Journal Entry: Ethical Dilemma 2

You are taking care of a 36-year-old patient from Vietnam, who has been diagnosed with a terminal illness. The family does not want the patient to know about her diagnosis, but in private the patient has asked you what her prognosis is. How do you handle this situation? What factors and ethical principles do you consider in your response to this ethical dilemma?

Your response should discuss the cultural and ethical dilemma posed by end-of-life decisions, including reference to the concepts of autonomy, beneficence, truth disclosure, informed consent, and family well-being. Your entry should be two to three pages.

Discuss your responses to this dilemma in small groups.

Works Cited

American Nurses Association (1980). *Nursing: A social policy statement.* Kansas City, MO: ANA.

American Psychiatric Association (2000). *Diagnostic and statistical manual of mental disorders (DSM-IV-TR)* (4th ed., text rev.). Washington, DC: APA.

American Psychological Association. (2003). APA Style.org. Retrieved January 25, 2006, from http://apastyle.apa.org

———. (2001). *Publication manual of the American Psychological Association* (5th ed.). Washington, DC: APA.

Bertrand, J., Seiber, E., & Escudero, G. (2001). Contraceptive dynamics in Guatemala. *International Family Planning Perspectives, 27,* 11–33.

Bosher, S. (2001a). Discipline-specific literacy in a second language: How ESL students learn to write successfully in a baccalaureate-degree nursing program. ERIC Clearinghouse on Reading, English, and Communication. *ERIC Document 454 707.*

———. (2001b). *Needs analysis of ESL baccalaureate-degree nursing students.* Final report, Project RN: Opportunity and Success. College of St. Catherine, St. Paul, MN.

———. (2006). ESL meets nursing: Developing an English for nursing course. In L. Kamhi-Stein & A. Snow (Eds.), *Developing a new course for adult language learners* (Vol. 5, TESOL Curriculum Development Series). Washington, DC: TESOL.

———. (forthcoming). *English for Nursing: Clinical Skills.* Ann Arbor: University of Michigan Press.

Bulmann, K., & McCourt, C. (2002). Somali refugee women's experiences of maternity care in west London: A case study. *Critical Public Health 12,* 365–380.

Calvillo, E. R., & Flaskerud, J. H. (1991). Review of literature on culture and pain of adults with focus on Mexican-Americans. *Journal of Transcultural Nursing* 2(2), 16–23.

Capps, L. L. (1999). Fright illness in Hmong children. *The Journal of Pediatric Nursing 25,* 378–383.

College of St. Catherine Libraries (2004). *Cultural assessment in nursing: A guide for locating resources.* St. Paul, MN: College of St. Catherine.

———. (2005). *Evaluating information found on the World Wide Web.* St. Paul, MN: College of St. Catherine.

———. (2006). *CINAHL: Cumulative index to nursing & allied health literature.* St. Paul, MN: College of St. Catherine.

Dorland's Illustrated Medical Dictionary (2000). Philadelphia: W.B. Saunders.

Gibeau, A. M. (1998). Female genital mutilation: When a cultural practice generates clinical and ethical dilemmas. *Journal of Obstetrics, Gynecologic, and Neonatal Nursing 27,* 85–91.

Giger, J. N., & Davidhizar, R. E. (1999). *Transcultural nursing: Assessment and intervention.* (3rd ed.). St. Louis, MO: Mosby.

Gold, S. (1992). Mental health and illness in Vietnamese refugees. *The Western Journal of Medicine 157*(3), 290–295.

Gordon, S. (1993, Jan.–Feb.). Caring means curing. *Utne Reader* 77–83.

———. (2000, February). Nurse, interrupted. *The American Prospect 11*(7), 79–88.

———. (1997, February). What nurses stand for. *The Atlantic Monthly 279,* 80–88.

Guthrie, C. (1999). Nurses' perceptions of sexuality relating to patient care. *Journal of Clinical Nursing 8*(3), 313–321.

Hales, A. (1996). West African beliefs about mental illness. *Perspectives in Psychiatric Care 32*(2), 23–30.

Hautman, M. A. (1976, October). Changing womanhood: Perimenopause among Filipina-Americans. *Journal of Obstetric, Gynecologic, and Neonatal Nursing 25,* 667–673.

Herberg, P. (2003). Theoretical foundations of transcultural nursing. In J. S. Boyle & M. M. Andrews (Eds.), *Transcultural concepts in nursing care* (pp. 3–65). Philadelphia: Lippincott Williams & Wilkins.

HighBeam Encyclopedia (2006). *Nursing—The modern profession.* Retrieved July 31, 2006, from http://www.encyclopedia.com

James, W. K., Smith, J., Kieke, B., & Wilcox, L. (1997). Female genital mutilation/female circumcision: Who is not at risk in the U.S.? *Public Health Reports 112,* 368–378.

Katz, J. R. (2001). Listening, memory, and test taking. In *Keys to nursing success* (pp. 205–230). Upper Saddle River, NJ: Prentice Hall.

Kimball, B., & O'Neil, E. (2001). The evolution of a crisis: Nursing in America. *Policy, Politics, & Nursing Practice* 2(3), 180–186.

Kozier, B., Erb, G., Berman, A., & Snyder, S. (2004a). Critical thinking and the nursing process. In *Fundamentals of nursing: Concepts, process, and practice* (7th ed.) (pp. 244–255). Upper Saddle River, NJ: Prentice Hall Health.

———. (2004b). Culture and heritage. In *Fundamentals of nursing: Concepts, process, and practice* (7th ed.) (pp. 205–222). Upper Saddle River, NJ: Prentice Hall Health.

———. (2004c). Historical and contemporary nursing practice. In *Fundamentals of nursing: Concepts, process, and practice* (7th ed., pp. 2–20). Upper Saddle River, NJ: Prentice Hall Health.

Kozier, B., Erb, G., Blair, K. & Wilkinson, J. (1995). Ethics and values. In A. Faulkner & D. Stahl (Eds.), *Reading strategies for nursing and allied health* (pp. 165–175). Boston: Houghton Mifflin.

Lapine, A., Wang-Cheng, R., Goldstein, M., Nooney, A., Lamb, G., & Derse, A. R. (2001). When cultures clash: Physician, patient, and family wishes in truth disclosure for dying patients. *Journal of Palliative Medicine 4,* 475–480.

Liamputhong, P. (2003). Abortion: It is for some women only! Hmong women's perceptions of abortion. *Health Care for Women International 24,* 230–241.

Longman advanced American dictionary (2000). Essex, UK: Pearson Education.

Matocha, L. K., & Waterhouse, J. K. (1993). Current nursing practice related to sexuality. *Research in Nursing & Health 16,* 371–378.

Mill, E. J. (2001). I am not a "Basa basa" woman: An explanatory model of HIV illness in Ghanaian women. *Clinical Nursing Research 10,* 254–273.

Miller, J. A. (1995). Caring for Cambodian refugees in the emergency department. *Journal of Emergency Nursing 21*(6), 498–501.

National Alliance on Mental Illness (1996–2007). What is mental illness: Mental illness facts. Retrieved September 28, 2007, from http://www.nami.org/content/navigationMenu/Inform_yourself

Reiff, M., & Zakut, H. (1999). Illness and treatment perceptions of Ethiopian immigrants and their doctors in Israel. *American Journal of Public Health 89,* 1814–1819.

Shives, L. R., & Isaacs, A. (2002). *Basic concepts of psychiatric-mental health nursing* (5th ed.). Philadelphia: Lippincott.

Steinbrook, R. (2002). Nursing in the crossfire. *New England Journal of Medicine 346*(22), 1757–1766.

Toubia, N. (1994). Female circumcision as a public health issue. *New England Journal of Medicine 331,* 712–716.

U.S. Census Bureau. (2004). *Immigrants admitted as permanent resident under refugee acts by country of birth: 1991 to 2002.* Retrieved January 24, 2005, from Statistical Abstract of the United States: 2004–2005 website, http://www.census.gov/prod/2004/pubs/04statab/pop.pdf

U.S. Census Bureau. (2004). *Immigrants by country of birth: 1981 to 2002.* Retrieved January 24, 2005, from Statistical Abstract of the United States: 2004–2005 website, http://www.census.gov/prod/2004/pubs/04statab/pop.pdf